D0262028

REVIEW OF MEDICAL HISTOLOGY

JACQUES POIRIER, M.D.

Associate Professor, University of Paris XII School of Medicine;
Section of Neuropathology of the Department of Pathology,
Hôpital Henri Mondor, Créteil, France

JEAN-LOUIS RIBADEAU DUMAS, M.D.

Associate Professor, University of Tours Faculty of Medicine;
Centre Hospitalo-Universitaire Bretonneau, Tours, France

translated by

URSULA TAUBE

edited and adapted by

PETER S. AMENTA, Ph.D.

Professor and Chairman, Department of Anatomy,
The Hahnemann Medical College, Philadelphia

W. B. Saunders Company / Philadelphia / London / Toronto

W. B. Saunders Company: West Washington Square
Philadelphia, Pa. 19105

1 St. Anne's Road
Eastbourne, East Sussex BN21 3UN, England

1 Goldthorne Avenue
Toronto, Ontario M8Z 5T9, Canada

Title of the original French language edition:
Abrégé D'Histologie
© Masson et Cie, Paris, France.

English translation published 1977 by W. B. Saunders Company, Philadelphia, London and Toronto

Review of Medical Histology ISBN 0-7216-7273-6

Print No.: 9 8 7 6 5 4 3 2

Foreword

Medical students no longer have enough curriculum time for detailed study of comparative vertebrate microscopic anatomy of tissues and organs. Although it is desirable, there is really no need for this. They must, however, have fundamental knowledge of the cells and tissues that function in the principal systems of the human body. A basic knowledge of the cellular and histophysiological processes is mandatory for comprehending the pathophysiology of most diseases.

The basis of our textbook is to present, in less than 250 pages, the essential histological information needed by a prospective physician. It seemed quite appropriate to present purely morphological data in tables or diagrams, and we preferred explaining, in text format, certain histophysiological information that was difficult to dissociate from pathological information. Texts, drawings, or diagrams are intended to complement, not duplicate, information.

Items of information which failed to point up significant physiological or pathophysiological facts were omitted. We have deliberately deleted technical details, esoteric discussions, and most authorities' names.

Part One, devoted to the cell, is considered solely to present basic information, not to be a review of the immense field of cellular biology.

Part Two is concerned with general histology, or the study of tissues. Those chapters dealing with blood cells and cells associated with immune responses or defense processes are more detailed because of their current significance in medicine.

Part Three treats of special histology, or that of systems. The nervous system is not included, since neurohistology, at least as it interests physicians, cannot be separated from neuroanatomy and neurophysiology.

We wish to express our gratitude to Mme. Isabelle Cohen, Chief of Histology-Embryology studies on the Medical Faculty of Créteil, who wrote the chapter on the female reproductive system, and who extended valuable advice.

We are deeply indebted to Professor J. Baudet as well as to Dr. J. M. Pelisse and Dr. J. P. Veron for their contributions in the preparation of this book.

Last but not least, we thank Mme. A. Feyfant for typing the manuscript.

J. Poirier
J.-L. Ribadeau Dumas

Preface

It is rarely an easy task to condense any subject matter, particularly when one must consider all component topics. Doctors Poirier and Ribadeau Dumas have been successful with the present text, which is geared to students of medicine and biology. They have abstracted the essential elements in the vast field of modern histology.

This text satisfies several needs: (1) it provides a valuable introduction to histology for medical and graduate students, and (2) during subsequent studies, it will provide a concise review of cellular and tissue structure. The complexity of modern medicine requires the student to constantly review basic material.

In addition to satisfying the needs of the student, this well-prepared review of current histological knowledge is invaluable for continuing education. Physicians and biologists who have found difficulty in keeping abreast of recent developments in histology will find this presentation extremely helpful.

Because of very strict requirements imposed in preparing any core text, it was necessary to be highly selective of material considered significant and relevant. In addition, since this book was intended primarily for medical students and those in allied fields, information that would provide a strong foundation for studies in pathology was emphasized.

Doctors Poirier and Ribadeau Dumas brought to this endeavor their valuable expertise gained from experiences as basic scientists and as clinicians. They surely deserve our gratitude for providing this well-written and valuable text, with its excellent diagrams and tables, which no doubt will render a great service in the study of histology.

RÉNÉ COUTEAUX
Professor of Cytology
University of Paris VI

Preface to the English Edition

The pleasant task of editing this first English edition was accepted on the conviction that it fills student needs in most Medical Histology courses. The concept of a core curriculum necessitates that material presented be critically selective and not merely reduced. The "core" should contain the "seeds" which, if properly planted, will grow to fruition in a well coordinated curriculum. All students should understand clearly that a core or review textbook, by its very nature, cannot take the place of the larger, more complete established texts. The core or review text serves to provide a busy student with an overview, and to stimulate interest in reading larger texts and, it is hoped, the literature cited in those texts.

Grateful acknowledgment is conveyed to Ms. Ursula Taube, who provided the initial translation. To Mr. Jack Hanley, Vice President and Health Sciences Editor of the W. B. Saunders Company, go my thanks for his patience, guidance and courtesies.

Special gratitude is offered to Ms. Mary V. Amenta for her many dedicated hours in typing, proofing, copy editing and preparing figures for the manuscript.

My faculty colleagues in the Department of Anatomy were particularly helpful. For their generous assistance in carrying on Departmental duties while this work was being completed, I am particularly grateful.

PETER S. AMENTA, PH.D.
Professor and Chairman
Department of Anatomy
Hahnemann Medical College

Contents

PART ONE THE CELL

PART TWO THE TISSUES

20

PART ONE
THE CELL

The cell is the smallest unit of living matter capable of independent existence and reproduction.

All cells that constitute tissues and organs are derived from a single cell: the fertilized ovum. Regardless of their degree of differentiation, they all possess certain fundamental characteristics which permit an independent existence. The specific characteristics of differentiation producing the many varieties of cellular specialization are discussed in Part Two *(The Tissues)*. In Part One, only those histophysiologic characteristics inherent in all cells are considered.

1

Cell Division

The majority of body cells in the adult (except nerve cells, which are not known to divide, and most muscle cells) have a limited life span, and can "survive" only by reproducing (cell division). This is an essential event leading to the formation of two cells from a single one. Each daughter cell receives all the genetic information encoded in the DNA molecules of the original cell's 46 chromosomes. This necessitates the duplication of the DNA of the "mother" cell and its equal distribution to the two daughter cells, so that each contains genetic material identical to that of the mother cell. Cell division, therefore, requires two successive stages: (1) *Biochemical* – duplication of DNA in the mother cell, and (2) *morphological* (or mitosis) – formation of two distinct daughter cells, each containing 46 chromosomes identical to those of the mother cell.

A. REPLICATION OF DNA

The coded genetic information is confined to the DNA molecules contained in the cell nucleus. The DNA molecule is composed of two chains wound helically around the same axis, and linked to each other via four complementary bases. Adenine links to thymine and cytosine links to guanine. As a result of this complementarity principle, if one of the two chains has the four bases in a certain sequence then the sequence of bases in the second chain will be determined as follows: Adenine will occur opposite thymine, cytosine opposite guanine, thymine opposite adenine, and guanine opposite cytosine. DNA synthesis, which can occur only by

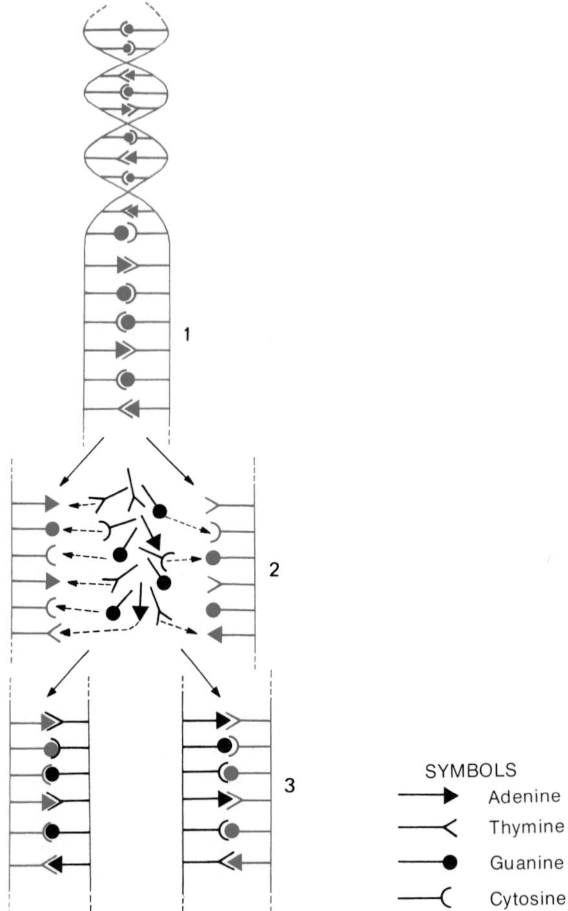

Figure 1. Duplication of the DNA molecule. *1*, A portion of the DNA molecule. *2*, The molecule splits into two parts, each possessing all the information required to reconstitute an entire molecule. *3*, Reconstitution of two molecules of DNA.

duplication of preexisting DNA molecules, produces an exact replica of DNA.

In effect the two chains of the molecule separate progressively and as their separation proceeds, each of the strands assembles the constituent bases in exact conformity to the principle of complementarity. The product is two molecules of DNA, each identical to the initial DNA molecule. In each of the two DNA molecules obtained, one strand originated from the initial DNA molecule, and the other is newly synthesized. This process requires the presence of an indispensable enzyme, DNA-polymerase, which carries out the course of DNA duplication before the morphological events of cell division become observable.

B. MITOSIS

Mitosis, a major upheaval within the cell, concerns mainly two types of structures: chromatin (which condenses into the chromosomes) and the centrosome.

I. Chromatin and Chromosomes

During the periods preceding mitosis, the essential genetic information is confined to the nucleus, where it exists in the form of tangled filaments of chromatin.

Each long and tortuous chromatin filament may be thought of as a single molecule of helical DNA encased in a protein sheath. Sequential duplication of DNA precedes the mitotic stages; the chromatin filaments

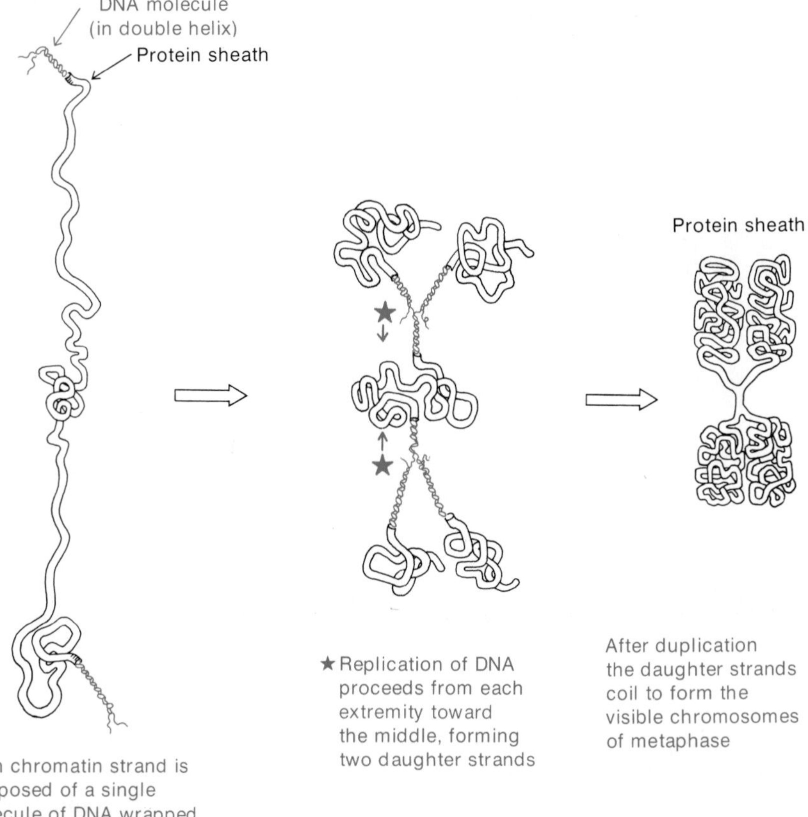

Figure 2. Model of the structure of chromosomes. (After E. J. Du Praw.)

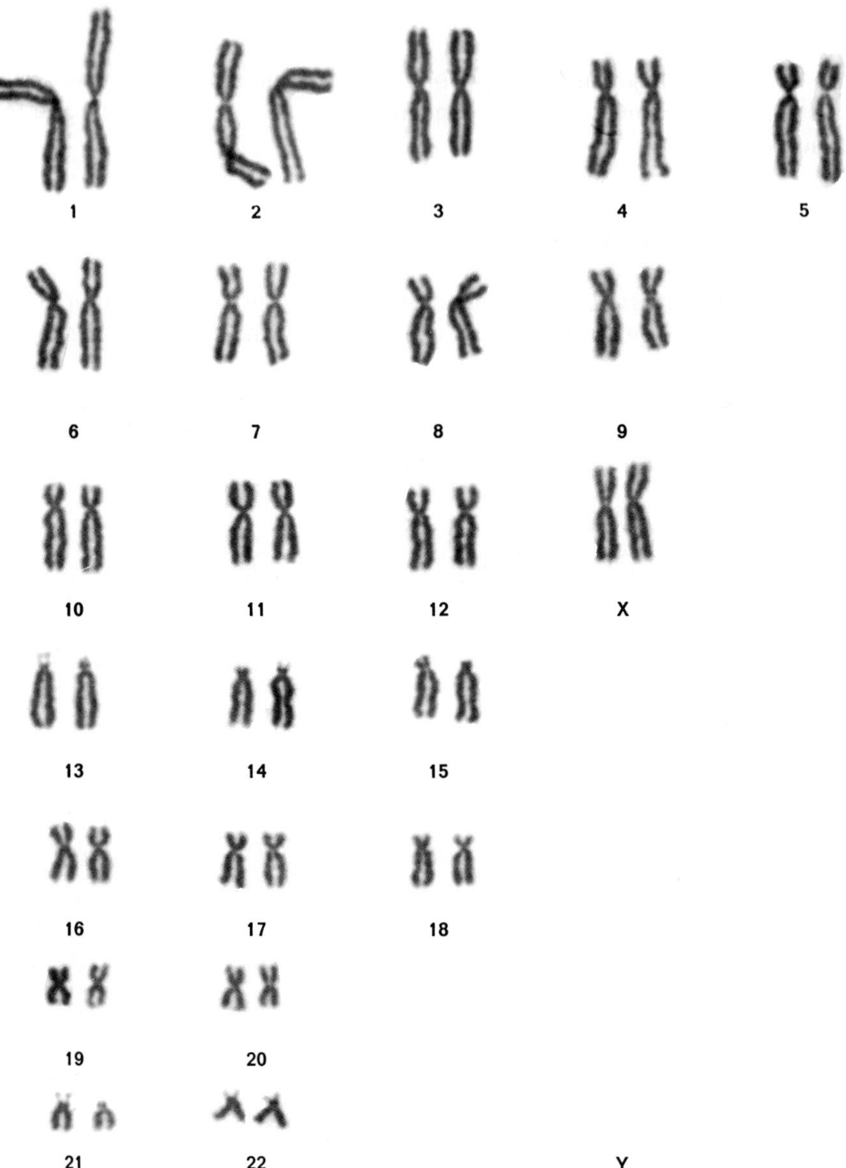

Figure 3. Karyotype of a normal female, arranged according to international nomenclature. Each chromosome appears as two strands joined by a centromere. (Photo courtesy of Dr. R. Berger.)

split lengthwise starting at the ends, and become coiled (due to the contractile protein sheath), producing the discrete metaphase chromosomes. The chromosomes thus become visible in the nucleus at the beginning of cell division and reach their maximum visibility at metaphase. The number and form of chromosomes are characteristic for each animal species. Chromo-

Figure 4. Schematic representation of mitosis in an ideal cell possessing only two chromosomes.

Interphase: The nucleus is surrounded by a nuclear membrane, which confines the chromatin and nucleolus. The centrosome, with its two centrioles, lies outside the nuclear membrane. *Prophase:* Granular chromatin appears as thin tangled filaments (*2*), which shorten and thicken (chromosomes). *3, 4,* The thickened limbs split longitudinally into chromatids attached at points called the centromeres (*5*). After some time, the nuclear membrane disappears; centrioles duplicate and migrate to opposite poles of the cell. Spindle fibers extend from one pole to the other between the centrioles, and chromosomes are attached to the fibers by their centromeres. *Metaphase:* Chromosomes arrive at the equatorial plate of the cell and arrange themselves in a radial fashion at the periphery of the spindle. *Anaphase:* The centromeres, which up to this time united the two chromatids of one chromosome, divide and liberate the chromatids, so that they migrate to opposite poles of the cell. (At this stage, each chromatid with its portion of the original centromere becomes a chromosome, with its own centromere). *Telophase:* The chromosomes assembled at each pole become less distinct and resemble the prophase stage (appearance of chromatin granules and disappearance of chromosomes). The mitotic spindle also disappears, and the cytoplasm constricts at the equatorial plate. Finally, the two daughter cells completely separate and resume the morphology of the interphase cell.

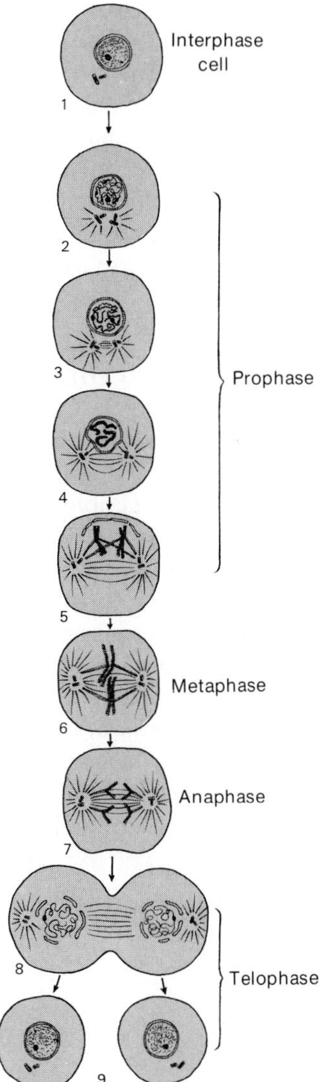

somes can be recognized and classified (karyotype) according to the length of the chromosomes and position of the centromere. In humans, each somatic cell possesses 23 pairs of chromosomes (46 chromosomes). Twenty-two pairs (numbered 1 to 22) are identical in males and females and constitute the autosomes. The twenty-third pair or gonosomes (sex chromosomes) differ for each sex: XX represents the female* and XY represents the male.

---

*In interphase somatic cells of the female, a small dark mass of chromatin attached to the nuclear membrane is observable with the light microscope. This mass, the sex chromatin or Barr body, represents one of the two X chromosomes, which is thought to be "inactivated."

II. Centrosome

The centrosome comprises two centrioles. Each centriole is a small hollow cylinder made up of 9 triplets of tubules lying parallel to one another and to the main central axis of the centriole. The two centrioles of the centrosome are oriented perpendicular to each other and in definite relationships to other microtubular structures of the cell—cytoplasmic microtubules, mitotic spindle, cilia, and flagella. The ultrastructure of basal corpuscles at the base of cilia is identical to that of the centrioles (see Fig. 14).

III. The Nucleolus

The nucleolus is a morphologically discrete organelle seen in the interphase nucleus. It is composed primarily of protein and ribonucleic acid (RNA), and functions as the site of synthesis for the principal components of cytoplasmic ribosomes. During interphase, nucleoli appear as dense, spherical structures via light microscopy and filamentous and granular via electron microscopy. Nucleoli are attached at secondary constrictions along the chromosomes. "Nucleolus organizing sites" thus represent loci at which information for RNA synthesis is encoded. Variations in number and size of nucleoli during interphase owing to nucleolar fusion and separation may reflect varying levels of ribosomal RNA synthesis.

Nucleoli "disappear" as discrete bodies during mitosis. The filamentous and granular material disperses along all the chromosomes at prophase and reaggregates during reconstruction at the "nucleolus organizing site."

2

The Interphase Cell

During the interphase period (between mitoses) the cell has frequently been referred to as being in a "resting state." This name is misleading, since nearly all metabolic and synthetic activity occurs during interphase. Indeed, whatever the cell's differentiation or specialization (glandular, mechanical, nervous activity, and so forth), its survival is due to continuous changes consisting of: (1) *synthesis* of its proper substance (structural and enzymatic proteins), (2) cellular *respiration* (supplying the necessary energy), and (3) intracellular *digestion* (entry, transformation, and discharge of materials).

The significance of cell membranes to cellular function justifies special consideration.

A. THE MEMBRANE SYSTEMS

I. General Structure

Most membranes possess common physical characteristics (i.e., thickness, surface tension, electrical resistance, capacitance, and water permeability).

In electron microscopic magnifications, sectioned membranes appear as two parallel black lines separated by a single lighter line. Numerous models have been proposed to illustrate the molecular structure of membranes. One of the more recent models ("fluid mosaic") visualizes a membrane with scattered globular proteins (or lipoproteins) embedded in a bimolecular layer of phospholipids (Fig. 5). The viscous nature of these

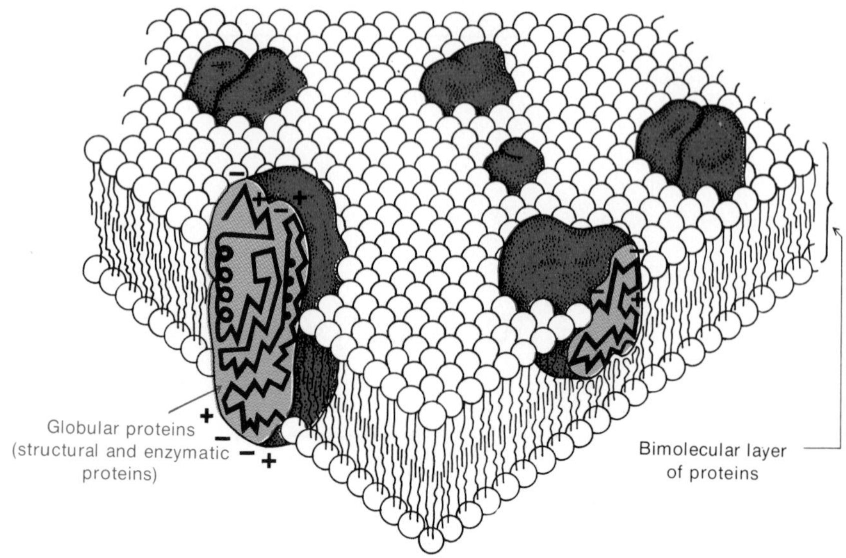

Figure 5. Model of the structure of membranes ("fluid mosaic" model). (After Singer and Nicholson, 1972.)

phospholipid layers is due primarily to the presence of unsaturated fatty acids possessing one or more double bonds.

On the external surface of the membrane is a protein polysaccharide coating (the "cell coat"), which is possibly secreted by the Golgi apparatus (or lamellar complex).

II. General Functions

Partitioning of Various Intracellular Compartments and Cell Limitations (see p. 11, *Distribution Within the Cell*).

Exchange. Membranes function fundamentally as a "barrier," controlling entrance and exit of water, electrolytes, and selected molecules at the cell level and in the various cellular compartments limited by the membranous systems.

Passive Diffusion. Diffusion across a membrane progresses very slowly for most molecules. Those which are more soluble in lipids penetrate more rapidly. Diffusion of *ions* is far more difficult than diffusion of *molecules,* since passage depends not only on a concentration gradient, but also on the electrical gradient within the system. Within the cell are large concentrations of *anions* which, owing to their size, cannot diffuse freely through the membrane. Under these conditions, diffusing *cations* and *anions* reach an equilibrium in which positive ions are more concentrated

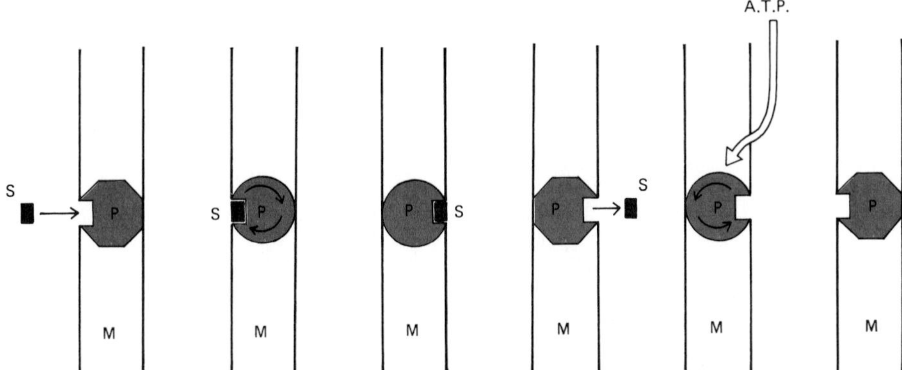

Figure 6. The permease system. The mechanism of active transport through membranes *(M)* may employ the system of permeases *(P)*, which captures the substance *(S)*. Attachment of a substance to the protein permease causes a change resulting in rotation of P. When S detaches from the protein and is released into the cell, the protein regains its original shape. Energy supplied by ATP causes rotation of the protein, allowing it to resume position and effect another transport. (After C. F. Fox, 1972.)

inside the cell than outside, and the negative ions are more concentrated outside than inside the cell. This equilibrium is dependent solely on physical forces, without any supply of energy by the cell. However, the existence of *active transport* modifies this balance.

Active Transport. Transport across the cell membrane necessitates expenditure of energy by the cell. The source of energy is ATP, produced by oxidative phosphorylation in mitochondria. Active transport may be effected by electrically charged pores. A pore might consist of the interstices between four adjacent protein subunits forming a hydrophilic canal through the membrane. Active transport of molecules may be performed by the systems of permeases (specific membrane proteins specializing in transportation).

Enzymatic Activities. Globular proteins that make up the membranes are either structural proteins or enzymatic proteins. The latter vary greatly, according to the nature of the membrane, and provide enzymatic functions of great importance for the cells.

III. Distribution Within the Cell

The Plasma (Cell) Membrane. The cell maintains contact with the rest of the organism through the plasma membrane which envelops the cytoplasm. Information is transmitted (membrane receptors, adenyl cyclase) and a variety of materials enter and exit the cell through it. Numerous enzymes are contained within the membrane, and antigens are embedded in its polysaccharide coat.

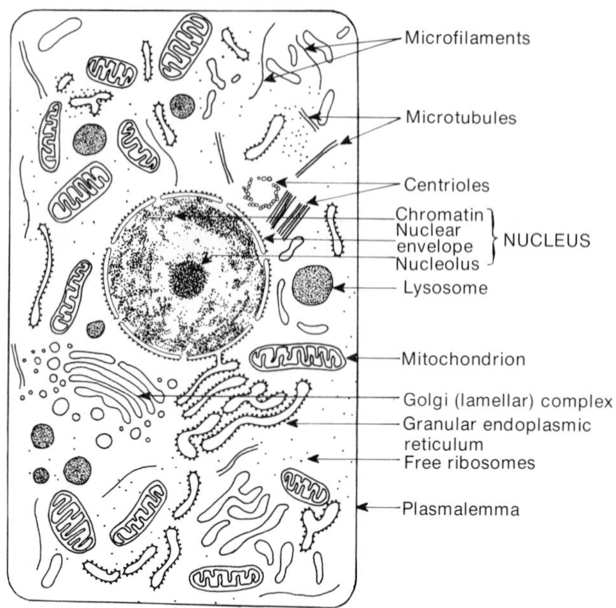

Figure 7. The typical cell as seen by electron microscopy.

Mitochondria. Mitochondria are bound by double membranes, which play a fundamental role in cell respiration (discussed in greater detail on p. 17).

Granular Endoplasmic (or Cytoplasmic) Reticulum. This organelle is an intercommunicating system of channels and cisternae bound by membranes with ribosomes adhering to the outer surface. These channels communicate with the perinuclear cisternae which form the "nuclear membrane." The cavity of this perinuclear envelope is continuous with that of the granular endoplasmic reticulum. The inner border of the nuclear membrane facing the nuclear chromatin is free of ribosomes; the outer surface may have attached ribosomes. This double (nuclear) membrane appears to be pierced by pores (inner and outer membranes being fused), which serve as an avenue for passage of materials between the nucleus and cytoplasm. The granular endoplasmic reticulum plays a fundamental role in protein secretion, and is therefore a characteristic feature of glandular cells which secrete proteins.

Smooth or Agranular Endoplasmic (Cytoplasmic) Reticulum. This type appears as a network of irregular tubules or cisternae bounded by a membrane. Ribosomes rarely adhere to these membranes. While occurring in all cells, it is most highly developed and characteristic of the following cells:

1. Steroid secreting cells: In these it participates in the synthesis of certain steroids.

2. Hepatocytes (liver cells): The smooth endoplasmic reticulum appears to play a role in enzyme degradation and elimination of liposoluble drugs, as well as in cholesterol metabolism.

3. Intestinal cells (enterocytes): The reticulum plays a role in the metabolism and transport of fats.

4. Parietal cells (in tubular glands of the stomach): In these it participates in production of H^+ and Cl^-.

Golgi Complex. The Golgi apparatus (or lamellar complex) occurs in all cells, but reaches highest development in protein secreting cells. It appears, via electron microscopy, as a stacked assembly of membrane-bound cavities, in the following forms: *saccules* (flattened and grouped like a stack of plates); *vesicles* (numerous spherules situated at the extremities of the saccules along their outer convex surfaces); and *vacuoles* (more voluminous spherules residing in the concavity of the saccules).

In addition to its fundamental function of protein secretion (formation of secretion granules in glandular epithelia) the *Golgi complex* plays an essential role in (1) elaboration of lysosomes (see p. 16), and (2) elaboration of glycoproteins and mucopolysaccharides (particularly those found in the cell coating).

Vacuoles. *The vacuolar apparatus* is a kind of intracellular digestive system comprising three types of membrane-bound granules: phagosomes, primary lysosomes, and secondary lysosomes (see p. 15).

B. PROTEIN SYNTHESIS

The vital fundamental task of each cell is the synthesis of its structural proteins and specific enzymatic proteins. Schematically, the process of protein biosynthesis results, at the ribosomal level, in an interchange of "information" from the nucleus and "building blocks" from the cytoplasm.

I. "Information" Component

The DNA molecules, which make up the chromatin filaments of the nucleus, carry the genetic information that determines the nature of the proteins synthesized by the cell. In effect the information on the specific nature and amino acid sequences of a protein are encoded in the DNA chains. The four bases (adenine coupled to thymine and cytosine coupled to guanine) making up the "rungs" of the "ladder" of the DNA double helix constitute this code. Each amino acid is determined by a known sequence of three bases. The order of these "triplets" or "codons" on the DNA helix determines the order in which the amino acids will assemble to

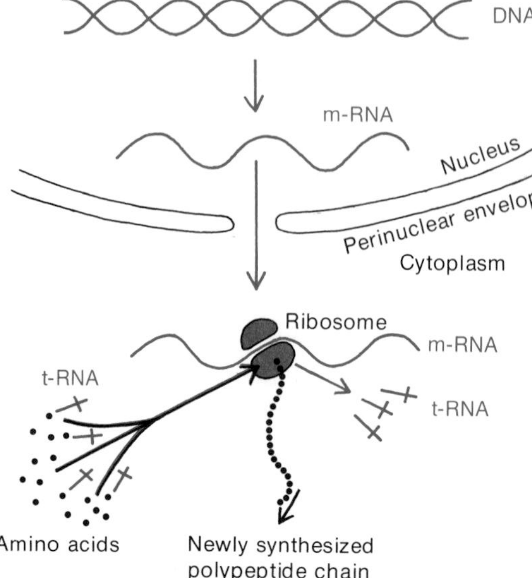

Figure 8. Protein synthesis.

form the produced protein. However, since the DNA molecules containing the genetic code cannot leave the nucleus, the code must therefore be transcribed onto an RNA (ribonucleic acid) molecule, which can traverse the cytoplasm. This type of RNA is called messenger RNA or m-RNA. RNA has four bases (adenine, uracil, cytosine, guanine) and the sequence of the four base types exactly reproduces the sequence of the corresponding bases of one of the two DNA chains (uracil is equivalent to thymine). These m-RNA molecules, carrying codons complementary to nuclear DNA codons, then attach to the ribosomes. The transcription process is dependent on the enzyme RNA polymerase.

II. "Building Blocks"

The building blocks of proteins are 20 different *amino acids,* which occur in the cytoplasm. Free amino acids are carried to the ribosomes by special RNA molecules designated as transfer RNA (t-RNA). Attachment of the amino acid to t-RNA is made possible by a specific enzyme, aminoacyl t-RNA synthetase.

III. Ribosomes

Ribosomes, the true protein synthesizing particles of the cell, constitute the sites at which m-RNA ("information" component) and t-RNA, with its attached amino acids ("building block" component), come together. The ribosomes *translate* information carried by the m-RNA and give it concrete form as a protein molecule of specific structure. The m-RNA traverses the ribosome, and codon after codon is read and translated from one end to the other. During passage of each codon triplet within the ribosome, the corresponding amino acid attached to t-RNA assumes its correct place. Additional amino acids progressively join and unite to form a polypeptide chain aided by the enzyme peptidyltransferase. Thus, the prescribed protein chain is formed and exits from the ribosome through a kind of tunnel.

Ribosomes, which are composed of ribosomal RNA and proteins, appear as small electron-dense grains under the electron microscope. Ribosomal RNA (r-RNA) is synthesized from DNA chains of the nucleus in the same way as m-RNA and t-RNA, but synthesis sites are grouped within the nucleoli.

IV. Control of Protein Synthesis

All cells of a given individual contain the same DNA molecules, and hence have identical genes. However, they do not all produce the same proteins, owing to the fact that not all cells translate the same DNA sequences. Certain sequences are "turned on" while others may be "turned off." Regulation of the activity of structural genes may be dependent on extrinsic factors (environment) or intrinsic factors (other genes such as operons or operator genes, and regulator genes).

C. INTRACELLULAR DIGESTION

I. Endocytosis and Exocytosis

In addition to passive diffusion and active transport, intake and elimination of materials by the cell occur by endocytosis and exocytosis. *Endocytosis* is the active entry of solid materials ("phagocytosis" means cell eating) into the cell by invagination of the cell membrane, which then would pinch off and be a membrane-bound structure (phagosome) within the cell. Pinocytosis (cell drinking) is the same process, except that the substance taken up is liquid rather than solid.

Exocytosis is the reverse process, resulting in the discharge of materials from the cell.

Endocytosis and exocytosis constitute two phases of intracellular digestion in which the *vacuolar apparatus* takes part.

II. Vacuolar Apparatus

Phagosomes contain material to be ingested, which is either of exogenous origin (heterophagic phagosomes) or of endogenous origin (autophagic phagosomes). They *do not* contain enzymes.

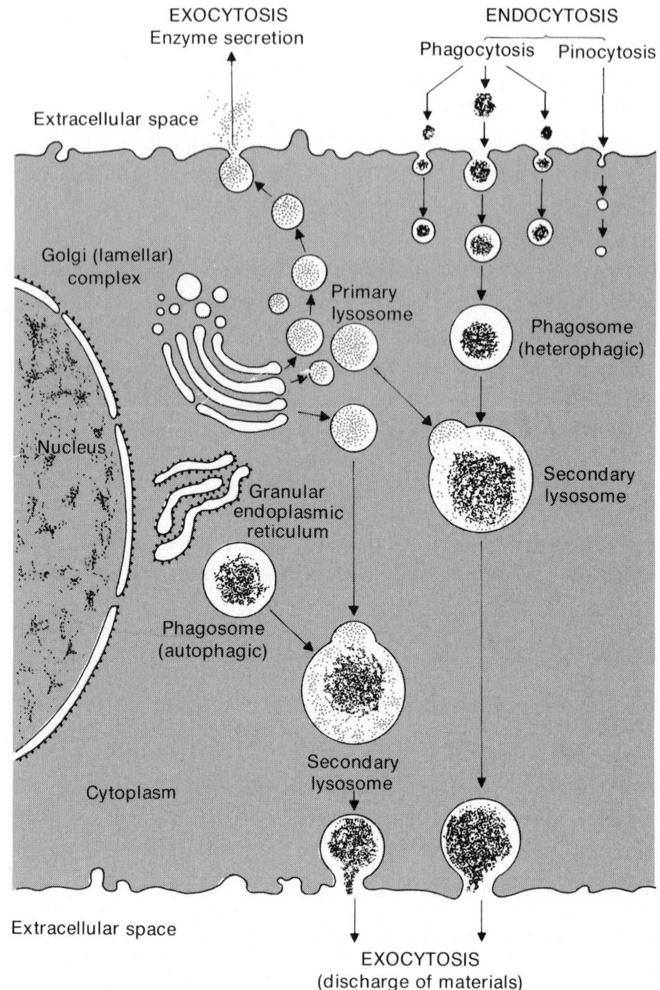

Figure 9. Vacuolar systems.

Primary lysosomes, formed by the Golgi complex, contain newly synthesized digestive enzymes (acid hydrolases) which have not yet participated in any digestive process.

Secondary lysosomes contain acid hydrolases and material being digested. They are called residual bodies when they no longer contain material other than enzymes and indigestible residues.

These three varieties of vacuoles are capable of performing exchanges *among themselves* (formation of secondary lysosomes by fusion of primary lysosomes with phagosomes); with the *outside of the cell* (formation of phagosomes by endocytosis of extrinsic substances; discharge of vacuolar contents by exocytosis); and *with the cytoplasm* (i.e., autophagy).

Because lysosomes play a most important role in the physiology of the cell, it is a fundamental prerequisite that the membrane enclosing this enzyme-filled sac be perfectly impermeable. If, under certain influences (ultraviolet irradiation, x-rays, ischemia, anoxia, bacterial endotoxins, and so forth), the membrane of the lysosome tears, the hydrolytic enzymes will spread throughout the cytoplasm to cause self-digestion (autolysis), which results in cell necrosis.

Lysosomes participate in numerous physiological processes. A few are listed:

1. Degradation of wastes from cellular metabolism.
2. Processes of senescence and natural death of cells.
3. Secretion of enzymes inside the cells (osteoclasts, enterocytes).
4. Cell division (opening of lysosomes could possibly initiate mitosis of cells that are prepared for division).
5. Defense against foreign bodies: bacteria, bacterial toxins, viruses, inert particles (these phenomena are mainly related to lysosomal activity of the polymorphonuclear leukocytes, acidophilic leukocytes, and macrophages).

D. CELLULAR RESPIRATION

Solar radiation is the ultimate energy source required by cells for life and for accomplishment of their various activities. Plants are autotrophic and can synthesize energy-filled reducing compounds from solar radiations, water, and atmospheric CO_2 (photosynthesis). Like all animals (which are heterotrophic), humans cannot utilize solar energy directly; they must absorb energy-filled reducing compounds synthesized by plants either directly (vegetable foods) or indirectly (animal food). Through oxidation of these energy-filled molecules (fats, carbohydrates, and proteins) the animal cell produces ATP (adenosine triphosphate), a form of immediately usable stored chemical energy. The reactions of intracellular respiration correspond to enzymatic reaction sequences and electron transfer which result in complete oxidation by atmospheric oxygen of carbohydrates, fats, and protein degradation products supplied by food. All these events occur in the mitochondria.

Mitochondria constitute an important part of the cell volume, and occur in variable numbers according to the cell type. They frequently appear to be distributed randomly within the cytoplasm; however, in certain specialized cells, mitochondria may be grouped in the active part of the cell. Electron micrographs of mitochondria reveal (1) an outer membrane, (2) an inner membrane forming folds or cristae, and (3) an amorphous matrix, in which dense granules are frequently observed.

Electron transfer occurs on the mitochondrial membranes (especially the cristae), while enzymes participating in the citric acid cycle (including lipolytic enzymes) are found in the matrix.

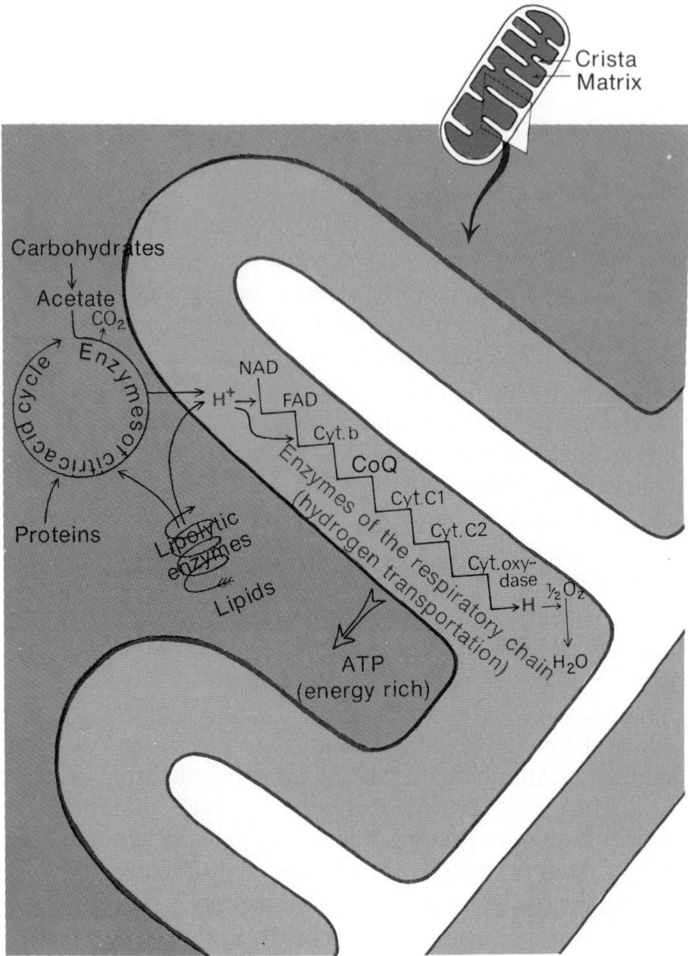

Figure 10. Mitochondria and cellular respiration.

Mitochondria possess a definite autonomy from the nucleus. They also contain DNA, RNA, glycogen, and proteins, and can multiply and perform protein synthesis. Some authors relate mitochondria to bacteria and believe they arose as symbiotic organisms of the cell, which during evolution became a permanent and indispensable component of the cytoplasm.

PART TWO
THE TISSUES

"A *tissue* is an aggregation of cells differentiated to perform the same function and grouped to that end in a certain order. . . . A particular tissue does not necessarily consist of identical elements, but of those elements which contribute to the same function. They may, indeed, present very different morphological aspects."

3

Epithelium

Layers of intimately apposed cells covering the external body surface and lining the lumina of various tubular organs and celomic cavities are termed epithelial tissues.

I. Intercellular Junctions. Epithelial cells are held together either by simple interdigitations or by complex membranous intercellular junctions. Little or no intercellular space exists between them, imparting a structural cohesiveness characteristic of epithelial tissues.

Intercellular junctions can be classified into several types, depending on how extensive in area the junctions are, and on how closely the membranes are apposed. In this regard, those junctions that are limited to a small disc-like surface are termed "maculae," whereas those that form a continuous band around the cell are called "zonulae." These two types can be further subdivided into maculae or zonulae *adherentes** (close junction) (in which a thin space exists between membranes), and maculae or zonulae *occludentes* (tight junction) (in which the membranes are closely apposed or even fused). In addition, plaques of varying size are sometimes found, in which there is less space between membranes than with maculae or zonulae adherentes, but the membranes are not fused (*nexus* or gap junction). In general, the most frequently observed structures are isolated maculae adherentes *(desmosomes)* and *junctional complexes,* consisting of three components (zonula occludens, zonula adherens, and macula adherens).

The permeability of the intercellular space may vary according to the type of junction system. In general, passages between epithelial cells are very tight. However, this cohesion does not exclude the presence of cells of different origin, such as lymphocytes, melanocytes, and nerve endings.

---

*Singular terms for these are macula, zonula, adherens, and occludens.

TABLE 1. Relations Between Epithelium and Connective Tissues—Terminology

Coverings			Epithelium		Subjacent Connective Tissue		Epithelium Plus Connective Tissue
Exterior surface of the body			Epidermis	+	Dermis	=	Skin
Body Cavities	Cavities open to the exterior (digestive tube, respiratory tract, and genital tracts)		Epithelium	+	Lamina propria	=	Mucosa
	Closed cavities	Celomic cavity (peritoneum, pericardium, pleurae)	Mesothelium	+	Submesothelial layer	=	Serosa
		Cardiovascular cavities	Endothelium	+	Subendothelial layer	=	Intima (for vessels) Endocardium (for heart)

II. Relationships with Connective Tissues

The lining epithelial cells are polarized. Their apical cell surfaces generally face the lumen of the organ, and the basal side is fastened to (or rests on) the underlying connective tissue by a "basal lamina." This latter structure consists of an extracellular layer of glycoprotein substances, rendered visible for light microscopy by special stains (PAS, silver). With the electron microscope it appears as a feltwork of ultrafine filaments.

The epithelia are devoid of vascular elements and are nourished by nutrients that filter through the basal lamina from underlying capillaries in the subjacent connective tissue.

Traditional names have been assigned to the various epithelia, subjacent connective tissue, and the epithelium—subjacent connective tissue complex, according to the kind of cavity they border (see Table 1).

III. Number of Cell Layers and Cell Shapes (Table 2)

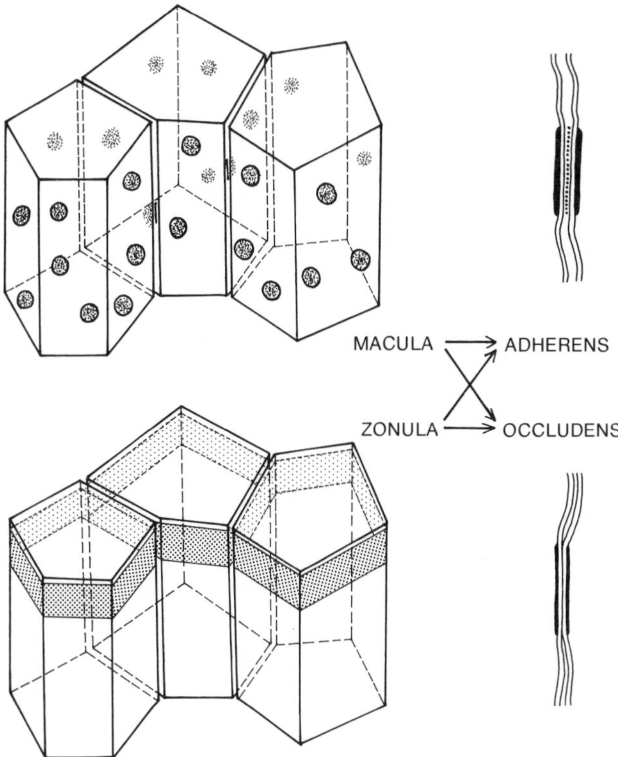

Figure 11. Principal intercellular junctions.

TABLE 2. Covering Epithelia

Number of Cell Layers / Cell Shape	Simple Epithelium (Single Layer of Cells)	Stratified Epithelium (Several Cell Layers)	Pseudostratified Epithelium (Nuclei Appear at Several Levels, But All Cells Rest on Basal Lamina)
Squamous Epithelium (Cells With Width Greater Than Height)	Simple squamous epithelium	Stratified squamous epithelium	
Cuboidal Epithelium (Cell Width Equal to Height)	Simple cuboidal epithelium	Stratified cuboidal epithelium	
Columnar Epithelium (Cell Height Greater Than Width)	Simple columnar epithelium	Stratified columnar epithelium	Pseudostratified columnar epithelium
Special Epithelium (Cells Have Forms That Are Too Different to be Classified With Above)	Visceral epithelium in glomerulus of the kidney	Epithelium of seminiferous tubules of the testes	Transitional epithelium of the urinary tract

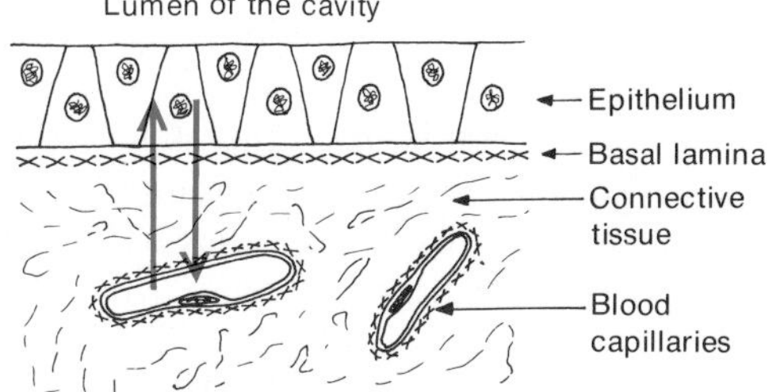

Figure 12. Relationships between epithelium and connective tissues.

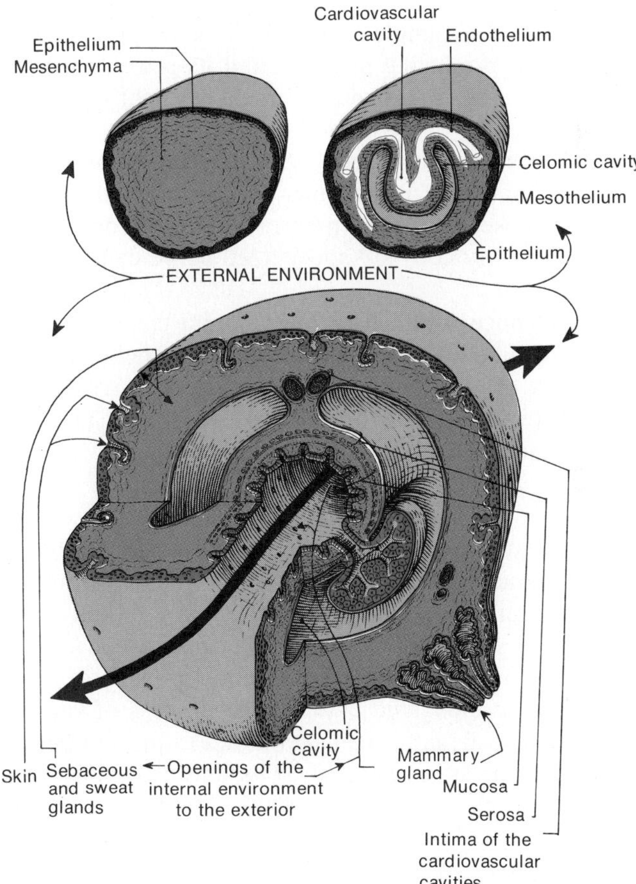

Figure 13. Relationships between the organism and the external milieu. (Redrawn after Elias and Pauly, 1966.)

IV. Cellular Differentiation and Functional Specialization

To perform their various functions (mechanical and/or chemical protection, movements, absorption, excretion, secretion, and sensory reception), epithelial tissues generally consist of specially differentiated cells. Their high degree of differentiation usually is associated with a relatively short life span. Cells are renewed by mitosis of undifferentiated epithelial cells (called replacement cells), which rest on the basal lamina.

Keratinized Cells. The accumulation of keratin is an inherent property of the most superficial cells of the epidermis (keratinized stratified squamous epithelium). Their main role is mechanical protection.

Pigment Cells. The simple cuboidal pigment epithelium of the retina is composed of cells producing melanin, and its primary role is protection of the light-sensitive rods and cones from excess light.

Sensory and Neurosensory Cells. Sensory reception in taste buds (in the tongue epithelium) and in the inner ear is provided by epithelial cells differentiated for those purposes. In certain sensory zones, such as the olfactory mucosa, sensory cells are specialized nerve cells.

Cells of Exchange Epithelia. Very important interchanges occur through simple squamous epithelia (vascular endothelium, mesothelium of serosa, epithelium of the thin loop of the nephron, respiratory alveolar epithelium). Their very thin cytoplasm is recognized in electron micrographs by the numerous pinocytotic vesicles.

Ciliated Cells. Ciliated cells make it possible for certain types of epithelia to propel substances within the luminal cavity bordered by them. These cells are characteristic of the respiratory and of portions of the reproductive tracts (efferent ducts, uterine tube). Ciliary motility is the result of the activity of very small contractile cytoplasmic appendages called *cilia.* The *ciliary apparatus* common to all cilia consists of three elements:

a. The *cilium,* an elongated cytoplasmic process of variable length, is covered by the plasmalemma (cell membrane), and contains an internal structure of tubules arranged parallel to its long axis. The tubules always possess the same number: nine pairs of tubules in a circle around the periphery, and two central tubules.

b. The *basal body,* which possesses a structure identical to that of the centrioles from which it derives; it is distinguished from the ciliary cross sections by its nine triplet tubules at the periphery without the two central tubules.

c. The *ciliary root,* a highly variable structure that emanates from the

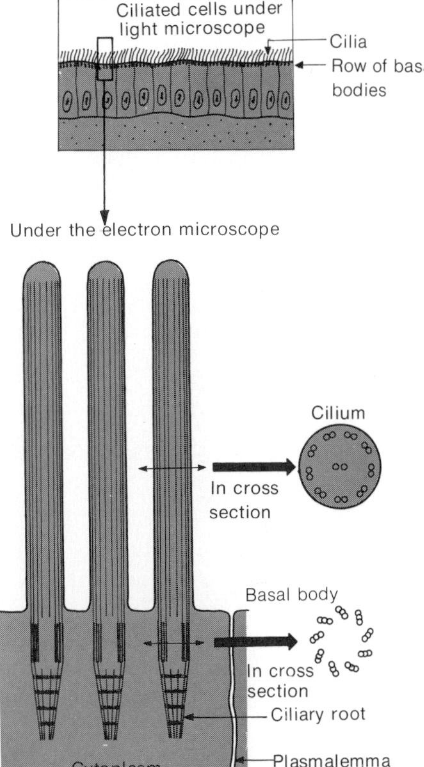

Figure 14. Morphology of cilia and basal bodies.

basal body and enters the cytoplasm. Although its functional significance is not entirely clear, it does appear to act as an anchor.

Ciliary motility may well work on the same basic principles as muscular contraction. Contractile proteins are present, some of which have ATPase activity, and the necessary energy source (ATP) is also present.

Glandular Cells. Some epithelia possess exocrine glandular cells (goblet mucous cells, gastric mucosal cells, and various secreting cells) and/or endocrine glandular cells (e.g., argentaffin cells of the digestive tract).

Cells with a Striated Border, Brush Border, or Stereocilia. Certain cells, specialized for absorption, reveal numerous microvilli at the luminal surface, whose precise organization varies for each type.

The three most important (see Fig. 15) are: (a) striated border in the intestinal epithelium; (b) brush border in proximal convoluted tubules of the nephron; and (c) stereocilia in the epididymis and ductus deferens.

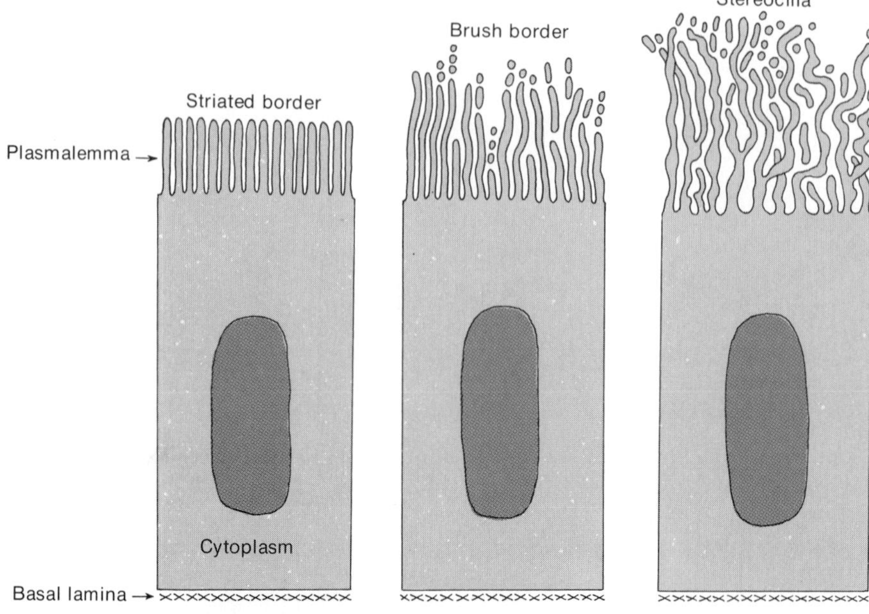

Figure 15. Principal differences in microvilli (specialized for absorption).

V. CLASSIFICATION

Epithelia are classified according to three characteristics—cell shape, number of cell layers, and cellular differentiations.

TABLE 3. Examples of Epithelia

SOME EXAMPLES OF EPITHELIA	CELL SHAPE	CELL LAYERS	SPECIALIZATION OF LUMINAL SURFACE
Stomach	Columnar	Simple	Short microvilli
Intestine	Columnar	Simple	Striated border (microvilli)
Trachea and Bronchi	Columnar	Pseudostratified	Ciliated
Epidermis	Squamous	Stratified	Keratinized
Vagina	Squamous	Stratified	Nonkeratinized

4

Glandular Epithelia

Glandular epithelial cells specialize in the elaboration of secretory products, which are released either into ducts (exocrine glands) or into the circulatory system (endocrine glands).

This cellular activity occurs in several stages: ingestion of materials required to manufacture the secretory products, synthesis of the secretory product, intracellular accumulation of the secretory product (in some types), and extrusion or expulsion of the secretory product.

Both exocrine and endocrine glands are derived from a proliferation of cells of an embryonic epithelium.

A. ENDOCRINE GLANDS

I. General Structure

The multicellular endocrine glands consist of glandular epithelial cells which in most cases are arranged in cords, bundles, or islets. A connective tissue stroma supporting the cell groups contains numerous fenestrated blood capillaries. The glandular cells of the thyroid have a characteristic follicular arrangement, whereas in some other organs, the endocrine cells may be scattered randomly.

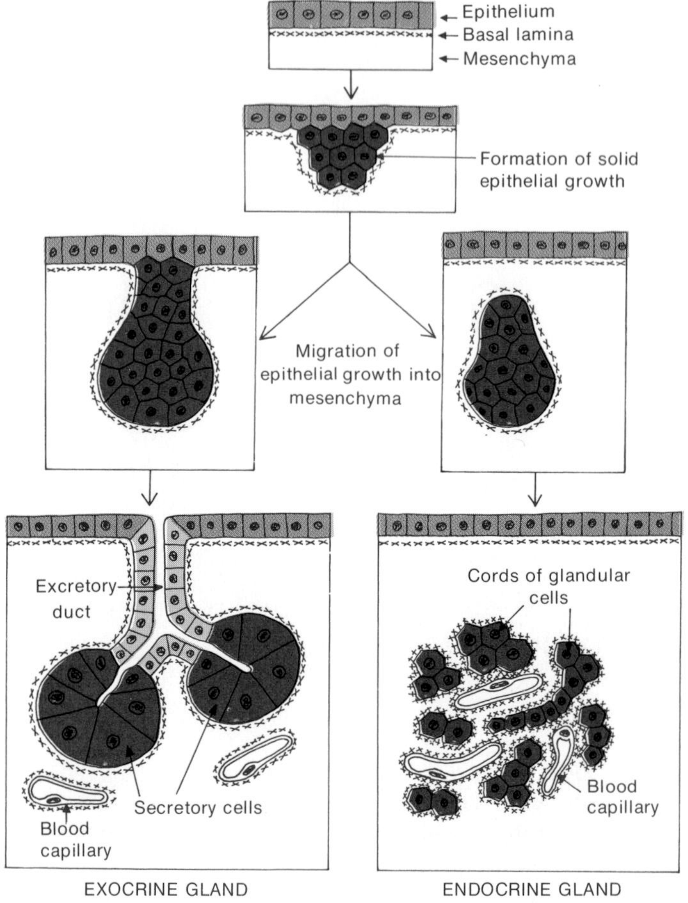

Figure 16. Histogenesis of glands.

II. Endocrine Glandular Secretion

Whatever the structure of the organs, the endocrine glandular cells always secrete hormones* directly into the neighboring blood capillaries. There are no functional excretory ducts in endocrine glands.

According to the chemical nature of the secreted hormone, four major groups of endocrine cells can be distinguished:

*A hormone is a specific chemical substance, secreted into the blood by a particular type of cell (endocrine glandular cells) and transported by the blood to a receiving organ (target organs) upon which the hormone acts.

a. Endocrine Cells Secreting Polypeptide or Pure Protein Hormones. The secretory mechanisms are as follows:

1. Proteins are synthesized by ribosomes associated with the granular endoplasmic reticulum from amino acids in the blood. This process is the same as that for the synthesis of structural proteins.
2. During synthesis, proteins enter the cisternae of the granular endoplasmic reticulum.
3. From there they move to the Golgi complex, where they are concentrated and packaged into secretory granules (where the secretory product is invested by a membrane of the Golgi complex).
4. The secretory granules, which pinch off the Golgi complex, migrate through the cytoplasm toward the plasmalemma, to which they adhere.
5. Finally, their contents are released to the exterior of the cell, by the process of exocytosis, and then enter the blood capillaries.

b. Endocrine Cells Secreting Glycoprotein Hormones. The cytophysiological mechanisms resemble those described above, but in addition, there is the inclusion of glycogen derivatives synthesized in the Golgi complex.

Because of these similar mechanisms, all endocrine cells involved in the secretion of polypeptides, pure proteins, and glycoproteins possess similar morphological characteristics: a distinct nucleolus, abundant granular endoplasmic reticulum, a well-developed Golgi complex, and membrane-bound secretory granules.

c. Endocrine Cells Secreting Steroid Hormones. The enzymes involved in synthesis of these hormones from cholesterol (drawn from the blood capillaries or more rarely synthesized in situ) are localized principally in the mitochondria (often with numerous tubular nonlamellar cristae) for some, and in the smooth endoplasmic reticulum or its vicinity for others.

The secretory product does not appear as a formed element, and the mechanisms of release are not well understood.

Steroid secreting endocrine cells have characteristic ultrastructural features: numerous mitochondria with cristae that frequently are tubular, extremely abundant smooth (agranular) endoplasmic reticulum, and absence of secretory granules. Lipid vacuoles (liposomes) resulting from accumulation of stored cholesterol esters (not from the secretory product) are frequently present. The role of these liposomes and lipoprotein pigments (lipofuscin) is not known.

d. Endocrine Cells Secreting Biogenic Amines. Enzymes involved in synthesis are located within the cytoplasm in some instances and within the secondary granules themselves in other instances. These always appear as small, dense-cored vesicles with the electron microscope. Their contents are released by exocytosis.

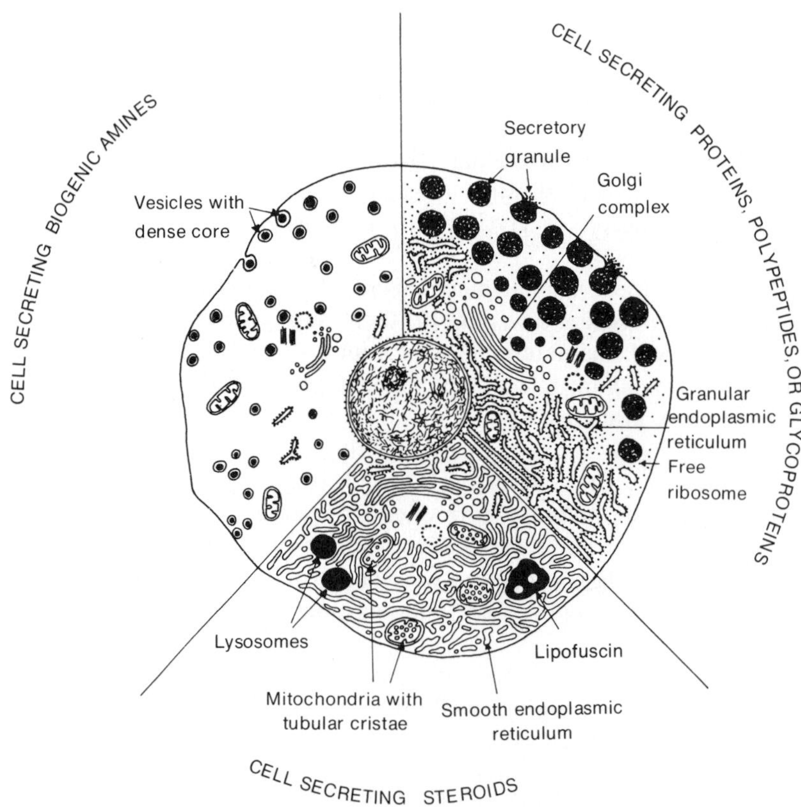

Figure 17. Schematic ultrastructural characteristics of the main secretory cell types.

TABLE 4. Endocrine Secretions

Anatomical Location	Endocrine Glandular Cells	Hormone Secreted	Nature of Secreted Hormone		
			Polypeptides, Proteins, or Glycoprotein	*Steroids*	*Biogenic Amines*
Adenohypophysis	Thyrotropic cells	TSH	+		
	Folliculotropic cells	FSH	+		
	Luteotropic cells	LH	+		
	Corticotropic cells	ACTH	+		
	Melanotropic cells	MSH	+		
	Somatotropic cells	STH	+		
	Prolactin cells	Prolactin	+		
Hypothalamus (neuro-secretory neurons)	Supraoptic nucleus	Oxytocin	+		
	Paraventricular nucleus	Vasopressin	+		
	Nucleus tuber	Releasing hormones	+		
Pineal	Pinealocytes	Melatonin			+

TABLE 4. *(Continued)*

Anatomical Location	Endocrine Glandular Cells	Hormone Secreted	Nature of Secreted Hormone		
			Polypeptides, Proteins, or Glycoprotein	*Steroids*	*Biogenic Amines*
Thyroid	Follicular	Triiodothyronine and thyroxin	+		
	C Cells	Calcitonin	+		
Parathyroid	Principal cells	Parathormone	+		
Adrenal cortex	Zona glomerulosa	Aldosterone		+	
	Zona fasciculata and reticularis	Glucocorticoids and androgens		+	
Adrenal medulla	Norepinephrine cells	Norepinephrine			+
	Epinephrine cells	Epinephrine			+
Pancreatic islets	B cells	Insulin	+		
	A_1 cells	Gastrin	+		
	A_2 cells (?)	Glucagon	+		
Testes	Interstitial cells	Androgens		+	

Ovaries	Follicular cells	Theca interna		Estrogen		+	
	Corpus luteum	Large lutein cells		Progesterone		+	
		Small lutein cells		Estrogen		+	
Juxtaglomerulus apparatus (kidney)		Juxtaglomerular myoepithelioid cells		Renin	+		
Digestive tube		Entero-chromaffin cells	Type I	Serotonin			+
			Types II + III	Enteroglucagon or secretin	+		
			Type IV	Norepinephrine			+
			Type V	Gastrin	+		
			Type V	Histamine			+
			?	Cholecystokinin	+		

B. EXOCRINE GLANDS

I. Morphology of Exocrine Glands

The general morphology of exocrine glands is more complicated than that of endocrine glands. Some lack an excretory duct and are composed only of isolated glandular cells, or of cells aggregated within an epithelium (intraepithelial glands, secretory epithelia). The majority of exocrine glands possess: (1) *a secretory portion* of glandular cells grouped as tubules, acini, or alveoli, and (2) *an excretory portion,* composed of an excretory duct, which may be unbranched or branched. Both secretory and excretory components are invested in a loose connective tissue stroma containing numerous *blood capillaries.* In compound exocrine glands (those with branched excretory ducts) the stroma demarcates lobules.

TABLE 5. Morphology of Exocrine Glands

Exocrine glands with excretory ducts	Excretory duct	Simple gland (unbranched) Compound gland (branched)
	Secretory portion	Tubular Acinar Alveolar
Exocrine glands without excretory ducts	Isolated glandular cells	Example: Mucous goblet cells 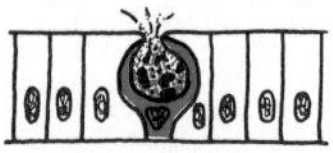
	Intraepithelial glands	Example: Urethral epithelium 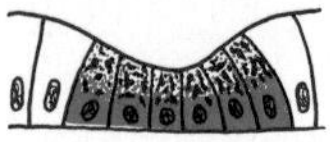
	Secretory epithelium	Example: Gastric mucosal cells 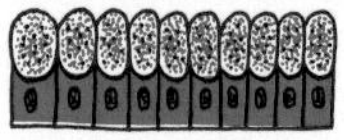

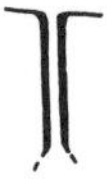

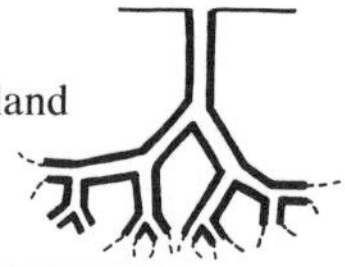

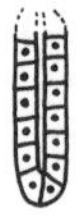

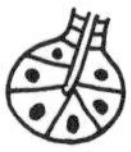

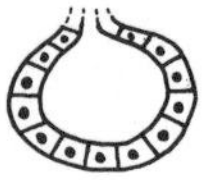

II. Exocrine Glandular Secretion

By definition, whatever the structure of the organs, the exocrine gland cells always synthesize a product to be released to the exterior (or skin), or into a tube corresponding to a prolongation of the exterior (digestive tract, respiratory tract, urogenital tract). The route might be direct (from cell to surface) or indirect, that is, by an intermediary excretory duct. (These glands are distinguished from endocrine glands in that the latter release their products directly into the *blood*.)

Depending on the chemical nature of the secretory product, several groups of exocrine glandular cells are distinguishable:

a. Exocrine Cells Secreting Pure Protein Products. These are the so-called "serous" cells (acinar cells of the pancreas and the parotid gland, the principal cells of the stomach, and so forth). The products they secrete are *enzymatic proteins* (trypsin, amylase, pepsin, and others). The mechanisms of synthesis, intracellular accumulation, and release are the same as those in endocrine cells secreting polypeptide or pure protein hormones.

b. Exocrine Cells Secreting Mucus. These correspond to the so-called "mucous"* cells (goblet cells, mucous neck cells of the gastric glands, and the myriad glands of the digestive tract, respiratory tree, and urogenital tract).

Mucus is a viscous product rich in mucopolysaccharides or mucoproteins. The processes of synthesis and release are the same as those in the endocrine cells secreting glycoprotein hormones. Usually the abundant mucous secretory granules cause these cells to appear "lighter" with the optical microscope than the "darker" serous cells.

c. Exocrine Cells. The cells of certain glands are specially suited to producing a particular secretory product and/or releasing it through a particular process of extrusion.

1. *Sebaceous gland* cells secrete a fatty product (sebum) onto the skin surface. The cells themselves, together with their contents, form the secretory product (holocrine gland).
2. *Mammary gland* cells secrete milk composed of two components: protein by exocytosis and lipid globules enveloped by plasmalemma (apocrine gland).
3. *Gastric gland* parietal cells secrete hydrochloric acid as Cl^- and H^+ ions, which traverse the plasmalemma. The plasmalemma, studded with microvilli, is invaginated in several points on the luminal surface as canaliculi.

---

*The secretory portions of some glands are wholly serous, others are wholly mucous, and still others are mixed seromucous.

5

Connective Tissue Proper

All connective tissues* are characterized by the presence of cells and fibers embedded in a ground substance. Several varieties are distinguished, based on the relative amounts of cells, fibers, and ground substance.

A. LOOSE CONNECTIVE TISSUE

Loose connective tissue has a wide distribution in the body and is part of the stroma of most organs. It is a major component of the mucosa and submucosa of the digestive tube, mucosa of the respiratory, urinary, and genital tracts, dermis of the skin, and submesothelial layer of the serosa. It plays an integral role in the constitution of peripheral nerves and muscles.

I. Basic Components: Fibroblasts, Collagenous and Elastic Fibers, and Ground Substance

Fibroblasts (or fibrocytes). Fibroblasts are fusiform or starlike cells with long cytoplasmic processes, which contain the usual complement of cellular organelles. With the optical microscope, the cytoplasm is indistinct, and the dominant feature is elongate ovoid nucleus with its one or two nucleoli. These fibroblasts synthesize the glycoprotein elements of the ground substance and the fibers.

*"Connective tissue" as used in this chapter does not include cartilage, bone, blood, hematopoietic or lymphoid tissues, although other authors do include these tissues under the very broad designation of connective tissue.

Fibers of the Connective Tissue

a. *Collagen fibers* are formed extracellularly from molecules of tropocollagen aligned end-to-end and side-to-side. Tropocollagen is synthesized and released as globules by the fibroblasts according to the previously described mechanism of protein secretion. (Tropocollagen molecules consist mainly of the amino acids glycine, hydroxyproline, and proline.) Via electron microscopy, collagen fibers are found to have a diameter ranging from 200 to 1000 Å, and reveal transverse striations at 640 Å intervals. These elementary fibers of indefinite length never anastomose and are often grouped in more or less wavy fascicles. If these fascicles are large, they are visible with the optical microscope, especially following treatment with special stains (they appear yellow with safronin, green or blue with the trichrome stains). These randomly oriented bundles or fascicles of the connective tissue stroma play an essential role in the mechanical support of an organ.

b. *Reticular fibers* are visible on silver staining as delicate anastomosing networks of fine black fibers. The term "argyrophilic" is frequently

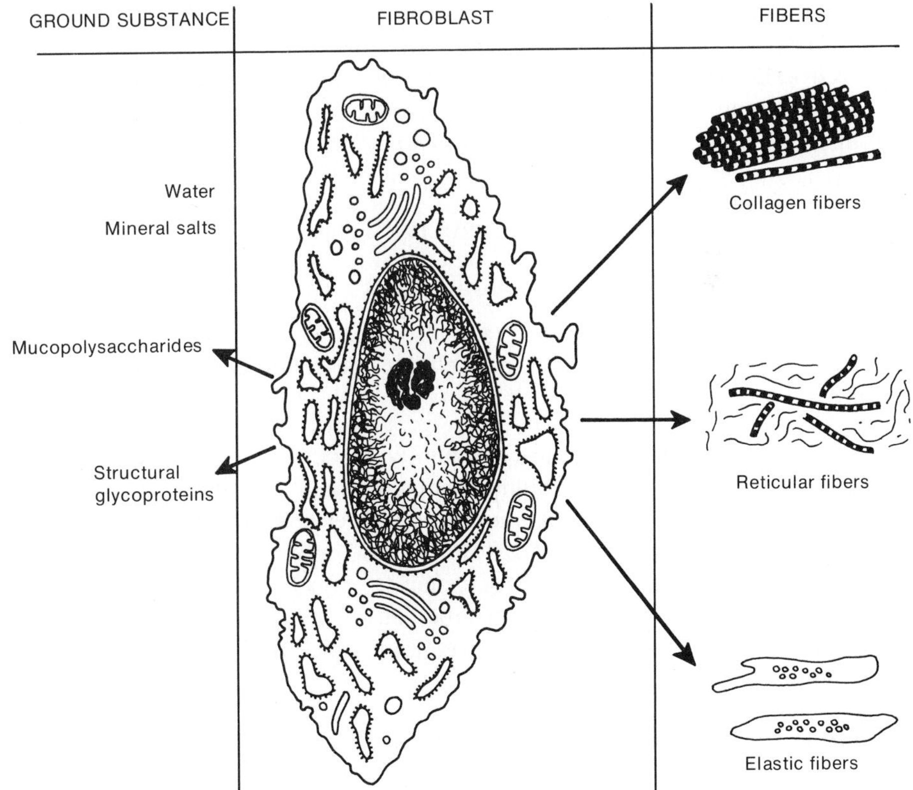

Figure 18. Basic elements of loose connective tissue.

used to designate affinity for silver stains. In electron micrographs these fibers appear identical to collagenous fibers of small diameter, dispersed in small numbers throughout the ground substance, but the reticular fibers may be made up of smaller aperiodic microfilaments (70 Å in diameter). They are found in normal loose connective tissue, but predominate in the reticular tissue of liver and the lymphoid and hematopoietic organs, where they are manufactured by reticular cells.

c. *Elastic fibers,* as their name implies, are characterized by elasticity, and are composed of certain amino acids elaborated by fibroblasts. The electron microscope reveals them as nonstriated microfibrils of a more or less dense amorphous substance. They can be rendered visible for optical microscopy by special staining with orcein or resorcin-fuchsin, with which they appear as a network of delicate, long, rather straight anastomosing fibers.

Ground Substance. Ground substance consists of water, mineral salts, mucopolysaccharides, and structural glycoproteins (closely related to collagenous fibers). These varieties of glycoproteins, like collagen and elastin, are secreted by fibroblasts. Ground substance can be stained for optic microscopy with PAS (periodic acid-Schiff reaction) and metachromatic stains (toluidine blue). Via electron microscopy, it appears as a flaky material of decreased electron density.

Ground substance plays a significant role in cellular nutrition, because of the exchanges taking place between the cells and the blood capillaries (found in abundance in connective tissues).

II. Cell Types in Loose Connective Tissue

Adipose Cells (see p. 41, *Adipose Tissue*)

Macrophages (or Histiocytes) (see also Chapter 6). These contribute, along with lymphocytes and plasma cells, to the defense role of loose connective tissue.

Mast Cells. Mast cells are frequently associated with small vessels. They are rounded cells containing metachromatic granules (visible with optical microscopy). Electron microscopy reveals these granules to have coiled lamellae. They synthesize and release into the ground substance (1) *heparin,* a sulfated mucopolysaccharide, known for its anticoagulant properties and its effect on the metabolism of lipids; (2) *hyaluronic acid,* a protein polysaccharide; and (3) *histamine,* which plays a role in allergic reactions.

Plasma Cells (see Chapter 7, *Lymphoid Tissue)*

Lymphocytes (see Chapter 7, *Lymphoid Tissue)*

Eosinophils (or Acidophils) (see Chapter 8)

TABLE 6. Dense Fibrous Connective Tissues

<table>
<tr><td>Irregular
(Fascicles of collagenous fibers intermingled in all directions with no specific orientation)</td><td colspan="2">Dermis
Periosteum
Perichondrium
Capsules (enveloping numerous organs)</td></tr>
<tr><td rowspan="4">Regular
(Fascicles of collagenous fibers arranged in regular, parallel manner)</td><td rowspan="2">With unilateral tension (fiber fascicles oriented in one direction only)</td><td>Ligaments (connecting bone to bone)</td></tr>
<tr><td>Tendons (connecting muscles to bones): parallel fascicles of collagenous fibers are enveloped in sheaths of loose connective tissue</td></tr>
<tr><td rowspan="2">With bilateral tension (fiber fascicles oriented in two directions)</td><td>Aponeurosis (connecting muscles to bones): made up of several anastomosed supraimposed layers of parallel collagenous fibers with orientations changing from one layer to the other</td></tr>
<tr><td>Stroma of the cornea</td></tr>
</table>

B. DENSE CONNECTIVE TISSUE

These tissues, serving mainly in mechanical support, are characterized by the (1) preponderance of fibers (collagen or elastic), (2) a few varieties of cells other than fibroblasts, and (3) a paucity of ground substance.

Dense Fibrous Connective Tissue. In this type, collagenous fibers predominate.

Elastic Tissue. Elastic fibers predominate in this type, which is found in larger arteries and ligamentum nuchae.

C. ADIPOSE TISSUE

Adipose tissue, in which adipose cells enclosed in a fine mesh of reticular fibers predominate, is found in hypodermis, retroperitoneal tissues, the mesentery, and the greater omentum. It contains numerous blood capillaries. The lipocytes (or adipose cells) are spherical and voluminous. Their nuclei are flattened or compressed by the lipid inclusion at the periphery of the cells. The cytoplasm is reduced to a thin sheet enveloping the lipid droplet but contains, nevertheless, the usual organelles, and in particular a Golgi complex and mitochondria. The lipids of the lipocytes are not static reserves, but are continually renewed, evincing an intense cellular metabolism.

The metabolic activity of lipocytes can be divided into three stages:

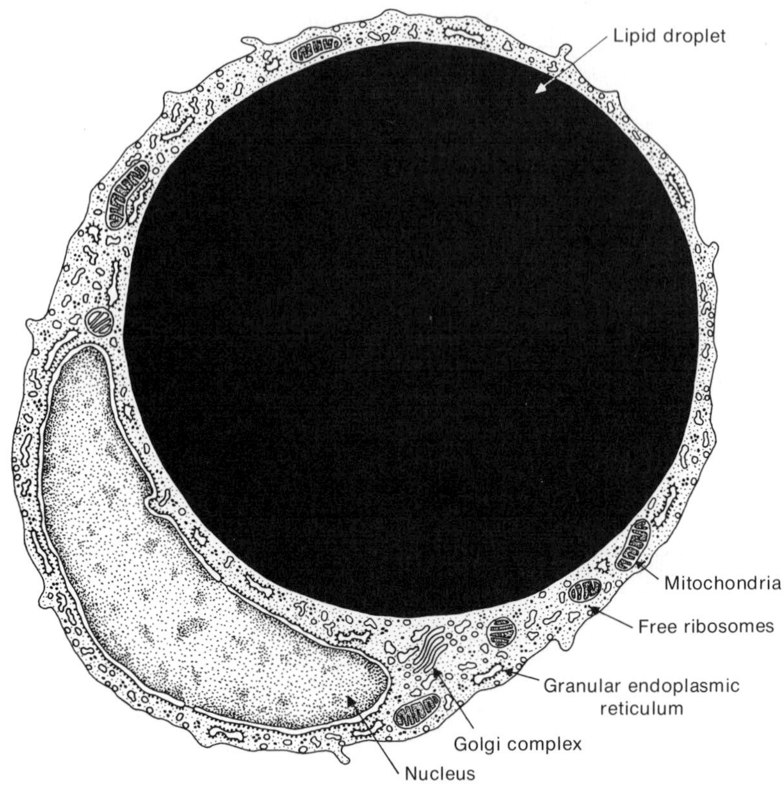

Figure 19. Schematic representation of a lipocyte as seen by electron microscopy. (From T. L. Lentz, 1971.)

1. *Synthesis* of lipids *(lipogenesis)* from different substrates (triglycerides originating in food and glucose).

2. *Storage* of lipids, as triglycerides.

3. Their release *(lipolysis),* especially as nonesterified fatty acids. The nonesterified fatty acids, which the lipocytes release into the blood, can be used by other cells as an energy source (either directly or after glycogenesis).

Thus, adipose tissue is one of the most important energy reserves which the body calls upon when carbohydrate reserves are exhausted (starvation, physical efforts, combating cold, and so forth) or become unusable (serious diabetes).

6

The Macrophage System

A. MACROPHAGES

Macrophages are mononuclear cells charged with clearing particulate matter from the blood, lymph, and other tissues (i.e., microorganisms or worn-out cells) by phagocytosis.

Cytoplasmic pseudopodia extend outward and draw foreign bodies into newly formed vacuoles (phagosomes). The numerous lysosomes contained in the macrophage release their hydrolytic enzymes into these vacuoles. The "treatment" of such particles within these phagolysosomes gives them a peculiar configuration (termed myelin figures). The macrophage encloses the ingested products and sometimes ejects them. It can also secrete hydrolytic enzymes into the surrounding ground substance.

Macrophages possess on their surfaces receptor sites for immunoglobulins and complement.

The life span of macrophages is calculated in weeks or months. In certain cases, they undergo a morphological evolution which causes them to progress through stages in which they appear as epithelioid cells and giant multinucleated cells.

B. THE MACROPHAGE SYSTEM

Macrophages are found in all tissues of the body. Two types are distinguished: fixed macrophages (proper to reticular tissue), and free macrophages (wandering cells).

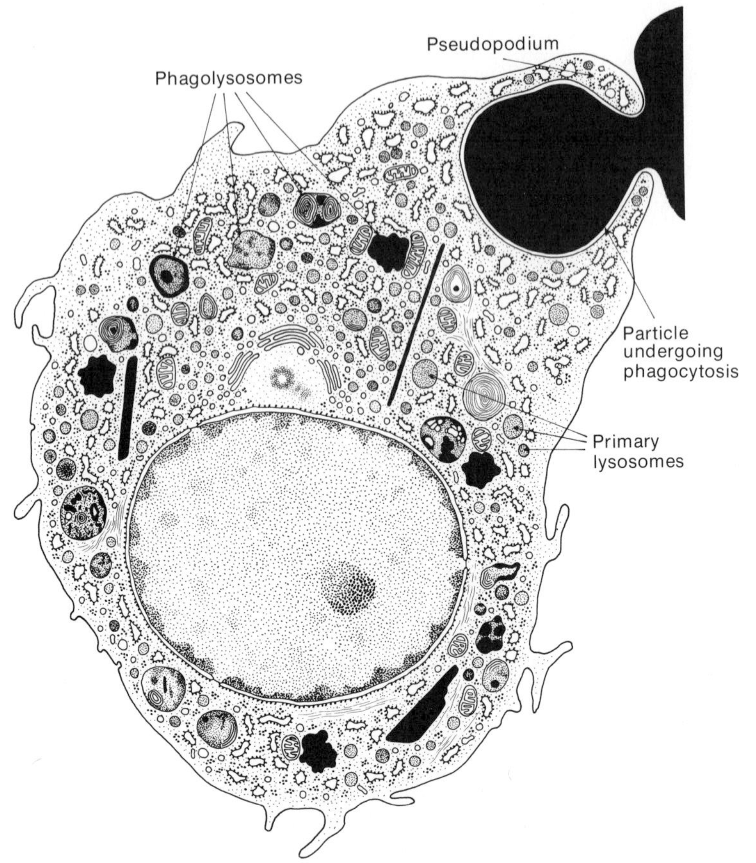

Figure 20. The macrophage as seen by electron microscopy. (Modified and redrawn after T. L. Lentz, 1971.)

I. Fixed Macrophages of the Reticular Tissue

Reticular connective tissue is composed of (1) reticular cells, with weak phagocytic potential; and (2) reticular fibers, which are elaborated by reticular cells and form a network to which these cells and their processes are attached.

In lymphoid organs (bone marrow, lymph nodes, spleen) the reticular tissue forms a fine three-dimensional network through which blood and/or lymph filters slowly. The reticular network thus gives structural support to the vascular filter constituting these organs.

The phagocytic capacity of reticular tissue is determined by its constituent macrophages: fixed macrophages (attached to the cytoplasmic processes of reticular cells, some of which form the walls of the blood and/or lymph sinusoidal capillaries) and free macrophages.

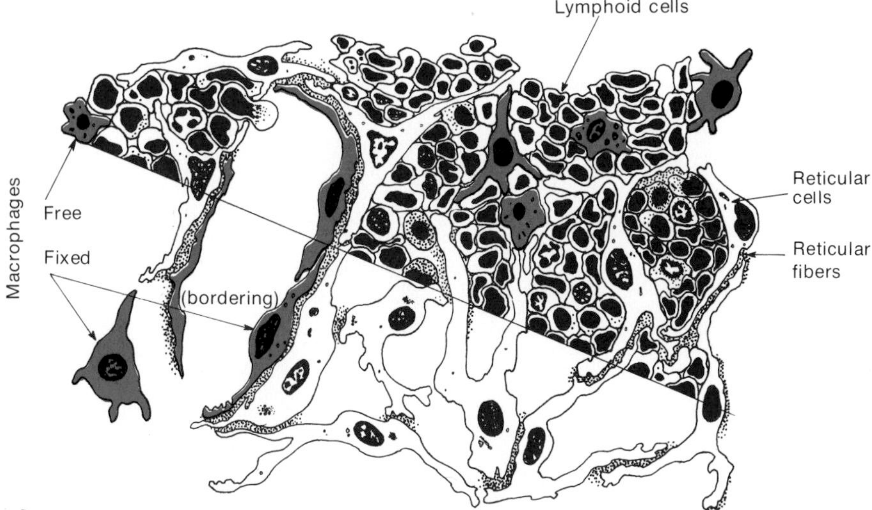

Figure 21. Reticular tissue. The reticular network of lymphoid organs is shown on the lower part of the drawing, and lymphoid elements contained in its meshes in the upper part. (After L. Weiss, 1972.)

II. Free Macrophages

Free macrophages are scattered throughout the body but wander predominantly within the reticular network of lymphoid organs, the alveoli of the lungs, and the connective tissues (especially the lamina propria of the mucosa and serosa).

Resting histiocytes (macrophages of the connective tissue) can hardly be distinguished from fibroblasts. However, when exerting their phagocytic potential, they display specific morphological aspects of the macrophages.

III. Origin of the Macrophages

Macrophages may be produced by mitosis of preexisting macrophages, or from blood monocytes, which are formed in the bone marrow from multipotential stem cells. The stages of differentiation and maturation are unknown, except for the promonocyte stage.

Monocytes are the immediate precursors of the macrophages, being, figuratively speaking, "forms of transport" capable of circulating in the body through blood, lymph, and connective spaces, to reach areas where macrophages are needed.

Macrophages and their precursors (stem cells, promonocytes, and monocytes) comprise the "mononuclear phagocytic system."

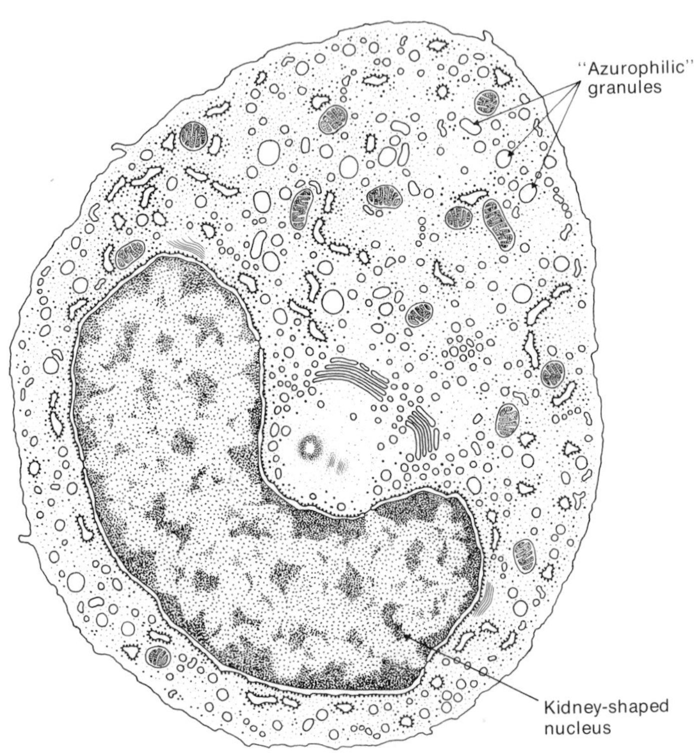

Figure 22. Monocyte as seen by electron microscopy. (After T. L. Lentz, 1971.)

TABLE 7. The Mononuclear Phagocytic System

Cells	Location
STEM CELLS ↓	Bone marrow
PROMONOCYTES ↓	Bone marrow
MONOCYTES ↓	Bone marrow, circulating blood
MACROPHAGES	Hematopoietic and lymphoid organs { Spleen, Lymph nodes, Bone marrow Liver (Kupffer cells) Connective tissue (histiocytes) Lungs (alveolar macrophages) Nervous system (microglia?)

IV. Migration of Macrophagic Cells

There is no clear distinction between fixed and free macrophages. Free macrophages depend on migratory movements. This is demonstrated by the passage of monocytes from bone marrow towards the connective tissues and their recirculation in the blood. Other movements have been demonstrated: from peritoneum to the deep abdominal lymph nodes, liver, spleen, alveoli of the lungs, and digestive tube. Migrations are relatively rapid and limited, as evidenced by the rarity of finding macrophages in the blood.

V. Defensive Function in the Organism

The diffuse organization of the macrophagic system provides evidence of its importance in the defense process.

1. *Mechanical defense.* Macrophages are responsible for the elimination of effete cells and foreign particles. Certain phagocytosed substances can be reused, and they contribute to the iron and protein cycles. Macrophages play a fundamental role in the process of scar formation and in bacterial infections where they eliminate breakdown products after the granulocytes have destroyed the bacteria.

2. *Immune defense.* There is close relationship between macrophages, lymphocytes, and plasma cells in the lymphoid organs. The reticular network is the site of their interaction, division, and differentiation. Previous exposure of the macrophages to antigen is of prime importance for the recognition of the antigen by cells with immunological competencies, and in turn by cells having roles in humoral and cellular immunity.

7

Lymphoid Tissue

The differentiation and maturation of lymphocytes and/or plasma cells occur in lymphoid tissues.

A. LYMPHOID CELLS

I. The Lymphocyte

Heterogeneity of the Lymphocytes. The lymphocyte, a mobile cell, generally lacks phagocytic ability and does not show morphological signs of specialization. Though structurally identical, lymphocytes represent a heterogeneous group of cells with different functional roles. They are separated into distinct lineages according to: (1) rate of division, (2) life span, (3) origin, and (4) immunological competence. As a matter of fact, they represent the central element of immunological capacities of the body. It is difficult to offer a formal classification; however, it is usual to associate T lymphocytes with a long life span and B lymphocytes with a short life span.*

Lymphopoiesis. It is possible that the lymphocytes originate from the hemocytoblasts (see Chapter 8, *Blood and Hematopoiesis*). From these, differentiation of the lymphoblasts might take place, which, through a more or less long maturation cycle, would give rise to lymphocytes. A most im-

---

*It must be kept in mind that numerous arguments indicate that hematopoietic stem cells have a lymphocytic morphology.

portant fact is that the small lymphocyte is not the final stage in the cell lineage but represents a state of temporary cessation in the continuing cycle of a new lymphocytic production. The division of small lymphocytes, easily induced *in vitro* by certain agents like phytohemagglutinin, is demonstrated by the blastemic transformation of the cell (enlargement, increase in the number of ribosomes, modifications of the nucleus). *In vivo,* the introduction or reintroduction of an antigen induces a transformation of lymphocytes with appropriate surface receptors and stimulates mitosis.

Lymphocytic Migration Currents. The lymphocytes follow complicated circulatory routes, which are important for the development, evolu-

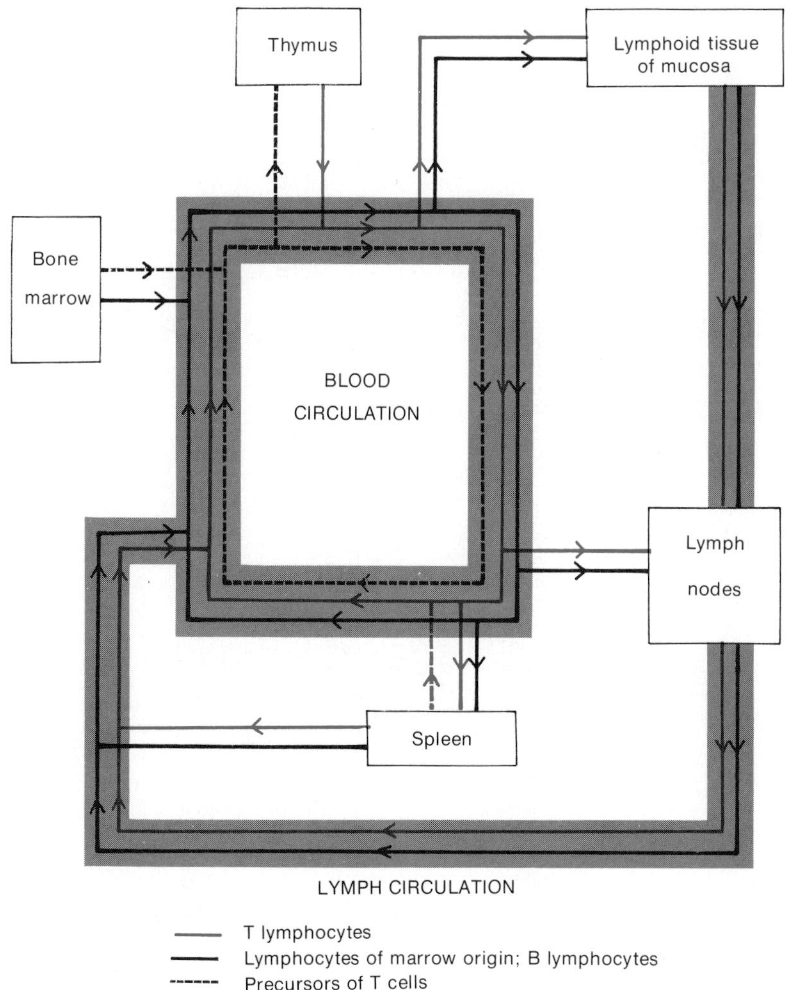

Figure 23. Circulation of lymphocytes in the organism.

TABLE 8. Classification of Lymphocytes

A. According to their immunological properties

	T Lymphocytes	B Lymphocytes
Origin	Thymus	Bone marrow
Distinct characteristics	Surface antigen θ	Surface immunoglobulins
Destination	Thymus-dependent areas of the organs and lymphoid tissues Periarterial lymphatic tube of the spleen Perinodular cortical area of lymph nodes	Medullary-dependent areas of organs and lymphoid tissues Medullary cords of the red pulp Medullary cords of lymph nodes Germinal centers
Role	Responsible for cellular events of delayed hypersensitivity Origin of lymphokines (substance affecting other cells, such as macrophages) Necessary for the recognition of antigens in the production of certain antibodies	Responsible for cellular events determining the synthesis of antibodies Can be transformed into plasma cells?

B. According to their life span

	Structure	Origin	Percentage in Lymphoid Tissues, Blood, and Lymph					
			Bone Marrow	*Thymus*	*Spleen*	*Lymph Nodes*	*Blood*	*Thoracic Duct*
Short life span (a few days)	Small, Medium, Large (lymphocytes)	All lymphoid organs	100%	95%	65%	35%	35%	10%
Long life span (a few months or years)	Small lymphocytes	Thymus (T lymphocytes)	0%	5%	35%	65%	65%	90%

tion, and distribution of immune responses in the organism. Schematically, stem cells (or undifferentiated lymphocytes) migrate from the bone marrow to the thymus, where they differentiate into T lymphocytes, which migrate into the blood and circulate between tissues and lymphatic vessels. They form a mobilizable and recirculating pool of immunocompetent cells. The B lymphocytes start in the marrow and colonize the peripheral lymphoid organs. They can recirculate with T lymphocytes.

Within lymphoid tissue, T and B lymphocytes can remain stable if they meet an appropriate antigen, proliferating and inducing the sequences of cell modifications of the cellular and humoral immunity.

II. The Plasma Cell

Antibody Production. The plasma cell synthesizes and secretes immunoglobulins by the same general process as protein secretion. Antibodies can be identified, via immunofluorescence, in the cisternae of granular

TABLE 9. Cells of the Lymphoid Tissue: Lymphocytes and Plasma Cells

	Lymphocyte	Plasma Cell
Morphology	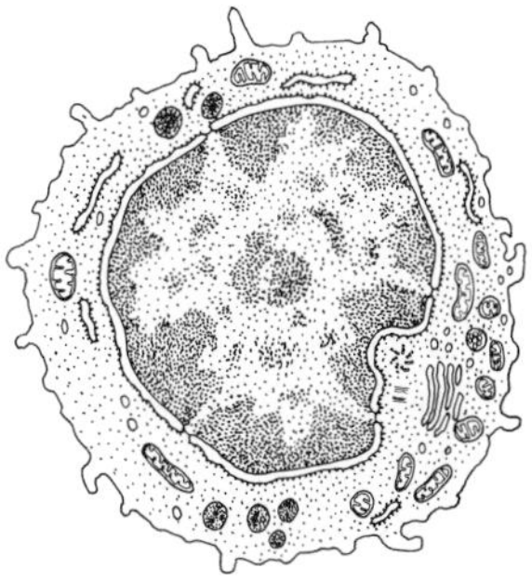	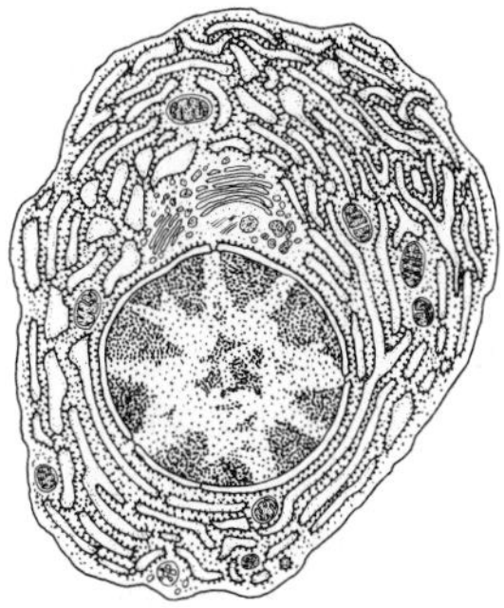
Diameter	5–8 μ = Small lymphocyte 8–12 μ = Medium lymphocyte 12–15 μ = Large lymphocyte	8–20 μ
Nucleus	Central Thick dense chromatin	Eccentric Chromatin arranged in cartwheel pattern
Cytoplasm	Reduced to a ring around the nucleus Basophilic, containing the usual organelles Sometimes dense granules	Basophilic (pyroninophil cell) Voluminous Golgi complex Abundant endoplasmic reticulum (sites of synthesis of antibodies)

endoplasmic reticulum. They often are greatly concentrated, and appear under the electron microscope as dense bodies surrounded by a membrane (Russell bodies).

Plasmacytopoiesis. It has been found that the plasma cell originates from a precursor, the plasmoblast, during the normal sequence of maturation. It is believed that maximum antibody production occurs during these transition stages. The mature cell is the fully differentiated terminal cell; the life span does not exceed a few weeks.

Antibody-producing cells originate in bone marrow. The stem cell appears to be the pluripotential cell with a less important differentiation capacity. Plasmacytopoiesis actually occurs in peripheral lymphoid organs. There are no plasma cells in blood or lymph, and only a few in the marrow.

III. Lymphocyte-Plasma Cell Relationships

Some small lymphocytes (B lymphocytes), in reaction to an antigen, transform and divide to yield a population of plasma cells or precursor cells. Some authors estimate that lymphocytes are capable of secreting antibodies. The problem is complicated further by the "lymphocytic" morphology that might be assumed by parts of the plasma cell lineage at certain moments of their life cycle.

B. ORGANIZATION OF LYMPHOID TISSUE

I. General Organization

Lymphoid tissue occurs discretely as lymphoid organs in bone marrow, thymus, lymph nodes, spleen, tonsils, Peyer's patches, and appendix, and diffusely in mucous membranes, especially those of the digestive tract, the bronchi, and the urinary tract. In all instances, except for the thymus (a very special lymphoid organ), lymphoid tissue always consists of a network of reticular tissue containing free macrophages and lymphoid cells. Thus, immune competencies determined by lymphoid elements are closely related to the properties of filtration-purification of the surrounding macrophage system.

II. Lymphoid Nodules

In lymphoid tissue, the cellular elements form a diffuse sheet. Except for the thymus, they gather within this sheet as lymphoid nodules, which are basic structural units of the lymphoid tissue.

The primary lymphoid nodule is a spherical mass composed of small lymphocytes.

The secondary lymphoid nodule has a peripheral ring of small lymphocytes and a lighter center, called the germinal center, formed by large lymphocytes, macrophages, plasma cells, and their precursors. Germinal centers are characterized by a large macrophage population and by an intense proliferative activity. The elaborated lymphocytes and/or plasma cells have a great capacity to migrate. The presence of germinal centers is closely related to the immunological competence of the lymphoid tissue. In the newborn animal, who has been sheltered from all antigenic contact, only primary nodules are found; isolated secondary nodules appear only after repeated antigenic stimulation. These germinal centers are antibody-producing structures, which become manifest at the same time as the secondary immune responses. They take an active part in the immune response and are rich in B lymphocytes.

8

Blood and Hematopoiesis

Blood is composed of cells suspended in a complex liquid, the plasma. Blood cells (which make up about 45 per cent of the total blood volume of an adult) comprise a cell population which is morphologically and functionally heterogeneous and undergoing perpetual turnover. Permanent cell interchanges occur between tissues and blood. Blood, therefore, can be considered as the principal vehicle for cell transport.

A. BLOOD CELLS

I. Red Blood Corpuscles or Erythrocytes

The erythrocyte is a highly differentiated cell responsible for maintaining the O_2-transport molecule hemoglobin, in a functional condition. The energy required for this function is derived from glucose contained in erythrocytes (intra-erythrocytic anaerobic glycolysis). The red corpuscle, an enucleated cell, cannot renew enzymes consumed in this intense metabolic activity, and eventually dies.

Its plasmalemma is coated with a polysaccharide layer containing antigens of genetic determination, which comprise diverse categories represented by many blood group systems, among them the blood types ABO and Rh factor.

II. White Blood Corpuscles or Leukocytes

These are nucleated cells, some of which possess distinguishing granules. They are categorized as follows:

1. Agranular Leukocytes. These comprise the lymphocytes and the monocytes.

2. Granular Leukocytes. These are mature cells, incapable of mitosis. They circulate in blood for a relatively short period, and within 12 hours, 50 per cent of the neutrophil polymorphonuclear cells exit the capillaries and enter the tissues, where, after functioning as phagocytes, they are destroyed.

Not all polymorphonuclear cells are in the circulation; they can be divided into: (1) circulating cells, and (2) marginal cells. In the latter group, polymorphonuclear cells adhere to the vascular endothelium, but, if needed, they are released into the circulation. The functions of eosinophils (acidophils) and basophils are poorly understood.

III. Blood Platelets

Aggregated in adhering clusters, platelets are fragments of megakaryocyte cytoplasm containing various organelles. They are rich in histocompatibility (HLA) antigens which play an important role in coagulation.

B. HEMATOPOIESIS

The constant disappearance of blood cells reflects a continual production of new cells. Most hematologists maintain that all blood cells originate from a pool of pluripotential stem cells (hemocytoblasts) which, when differentiated and matured into adult forms, are morphologically and functionally distinct. Division and subsequent maturation of cells occur exponentially.

In the adult, hematopoiesis normally occurs in bone marrow, except that the lymphocytes are produced in lymphatic tissues as well. When bone marrow has been destroyed by irradiation only marrow transplant can correct the situation, proving that stem cells originate in bone marrow.

I. The Maturation of Blood Cell Lineages

All cells developing toward the final adult stage constitute a distinct cell lineage. The various morphological forms are transitory stages as cells progressively differentiate towards their final form.

TABLE 10. Blood Cells: Erythrocytes, Polymorphonuclear Cells, Platelets

		Erythrocytes	Granulocytes	Platelets
STRUCTURE	Diameter	7.5 μ	9–14 μ	1.5–2 μ
	Shape	Biconcave disc	Variable	Flattened
	Nucleus	No nucleus	Several lobes (polymorphonuclear)	No nucleus
	Cytoplasm	No organelles Red pigment—*hemoglobin* (1/3 of the weight)	Usual organelles Special granulation according to the variety of polymorphonuclear cell (See Table 11)	Colored granulations, chromomeres Some cellular inclusions
FUNCTIONS AND PROPERTIES		Responsible for: transport and proper functioning of hemoglobin (the respiratory pigment which transports O_2 and CO_2)	Motility (ameboid): pass through endothelium (diapedesis); attracted by certain substances (chemotaxis) Phagocytosis	Protect vascular endothelium Primary hemostasis (assists in clotting) Synthesis of thrombosthenin (retraction of the clot)
DESTINY	Life span	120 days	Several days?	8–12 days
	Site of destruction	Bone marrow; spleen	Tissues of body	Liver and spleen

TABLE 11. Blood Cells: Granulocytes

		Neutrophilic Polymorphonuclear Cells	Eosinophilic Polymorphonuclear Cells	Basophilic Polymorphonuclear Cells
ELECTRON MICROSCOPE DIAGRAM		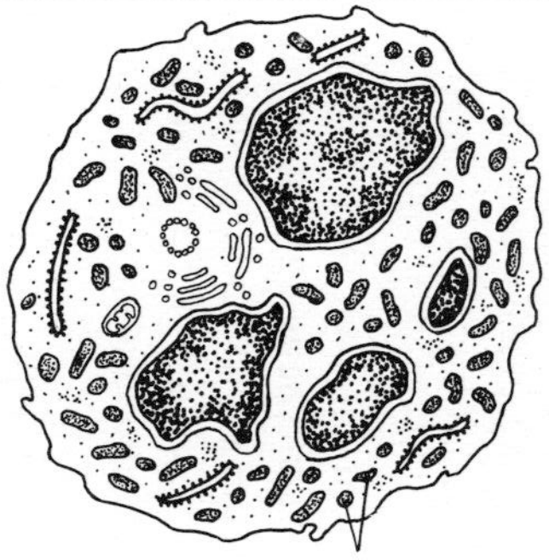 Primary lysosomes ("neutrophilic" granulations)	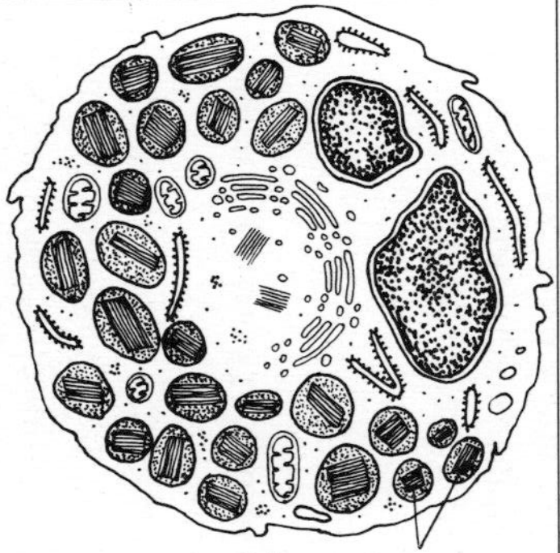 Primary lysosomes ("eosinophilic" granulations)	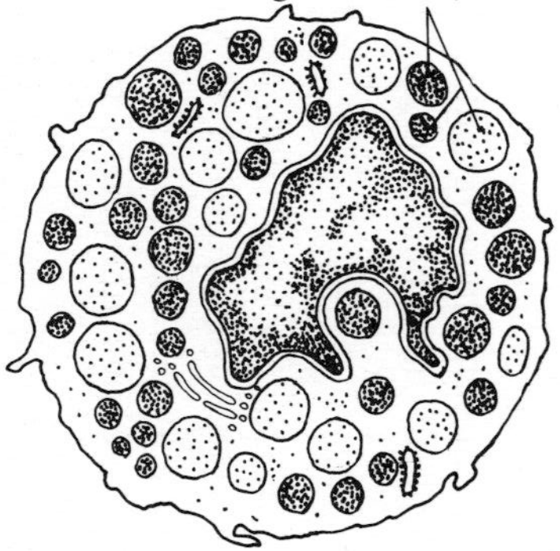 Primary lysosomes ("basophilic" granulations)
PERCENTAGE OF LEUKOCYTES		65–80	2–4	0.5–1
NUCLEUS		Several lobes connected by narrow strands of chromatin	Two to three lobes connected by a thick bridge of chromatin	Irregular, horseshoe-shaped
GRANULES (PRIMARY LYSOSOMES)	Optical Microscope	Small, regularly distributed	Large, rounded, refractile, red-colored	Variable in size, metachromatic (staining red with toluidine blue)
	Electron Microscope	Membrane-bound granules	Granules have central crystalline structure	Cluster of dense membrane-bound granules
FUNCTIONS		Phagocytosis of foreign bodies; antibacterial defense	Phagocytosis of the antigen-antibody complexes; transport and synthesis of plasminogen?	Role in delayed hypersensitivity

Erythrocytic Lineage. The process of maturation of erythrocytes is well known from demonstrations via radioactive labeling. The process commences with the synthesis of hemoglobin in the proerythroblast. During further evolution, the nuclear material is condensed, and its subsequent expulsion from the cell results in the enucleate reticulocyte. Hemoglobin continues to be synthesized until all intracellular organelles completely disappear.

Granulocytic Lineage. Differentiation starts with the myeloblast, a cell containing abundant material for protein synthesis. Continued differentiation is characterized by decrease in cell size, nuclear segmentation, and granular differentiation. The cells divide until they reach the metamyelocytic stage.

Platelet Lineage. Cell amplification takes place with a succession of nuclear DNA replications without cytoplasmic division. Partitioning of the megakaryocytic cytoplasm gives rise to a great number of platelets (up to 2000), which are released into the blood.

II. The Stem Cell and the Differentiation Process

Pluripotential Stem Cell (Hemocytoblast). When hematopoietic tissue is experimentally destroyed by radiation, it can be reconstituted by transplantation of marrow cells from another animal (of the same species). Several days following the transplantation, cell nodules appear in the spleen. These are formed by colonies of hematopoietic cells, derived from a single cell clone, or CFU (Colony Forming Unit). One CFU can restart the entire hematopoietic and lymphoid system.

Kinetic studies of the CFU show that they are self-perpetuating. The cell pool remains constant, indicating that the hemocytoblast is, in a certain sense, immortal. Unlike other cells of the hematopoietic system, they do not actively proliferate, and 80 to 90 per cent are in the resting state. They become active only if a peripheral cellular need arises (i.e., hemorrhage).

Differentiation of Stem Cells: Precursor Cells. There exist in the bone marrow "precursor" cells that constitute the intermediary stage between the stem cells and the fully differentiated cells. These are the cells which are most active in any cell line.

Red Blood Cell Lineage. The ERC (erythropoietin responsive cell) is a precursor cell which, by a plasma factor, erythropoietin, can be induced to differentiate towards the proerythroblast. A descendent of the CFU, it is an actively proliferating transitory cell undergoing maturation (pre-ERC is insensitive to erythropoietin and ERC is sensitive to its action).

TABLE 12. Blood Count in the Normal Adult

ERYTHROCYTES	4.5 to 5 million per mm^3 of blood			
LEUKOCYTES	6000 to 8000 per mm^3 of blood	POLYMORPHONUCLEAR CELLS	Neutrophils	60 to 65%
			Acidophils	1 to 2%
			Basophils	0.5 to 1%
		LYMPHOCYTES		25 to 30%
		MONOCYTES		6 to 8%
PLATELETS	200,000 to 300,000 per mm^3 of blood			

Granulocytic Lineage. Marrow cells, cultured on a semisolid gel, develop cell colonies of granulocytic lineage. These *in vitro* colony forming cells or ACU (Agar Colony Unit) could be the precursor cells of the white cell lineage similar to the ERC.

Other Lineages. The mechanisms of differentiation for these are unknown. It is uncertain whether intermediate precursors exist between the pluripotential stem cell and the lymphoblast.

III. Cell Compartmentations During Hematopoiesis

The hematopoietic system is formed of several cell foci having different functional and proliferative activities.

Stem Cell Compartment (CFU). These cells are pluripotential; for the most part they do not form part of the normal cell line but do so when the

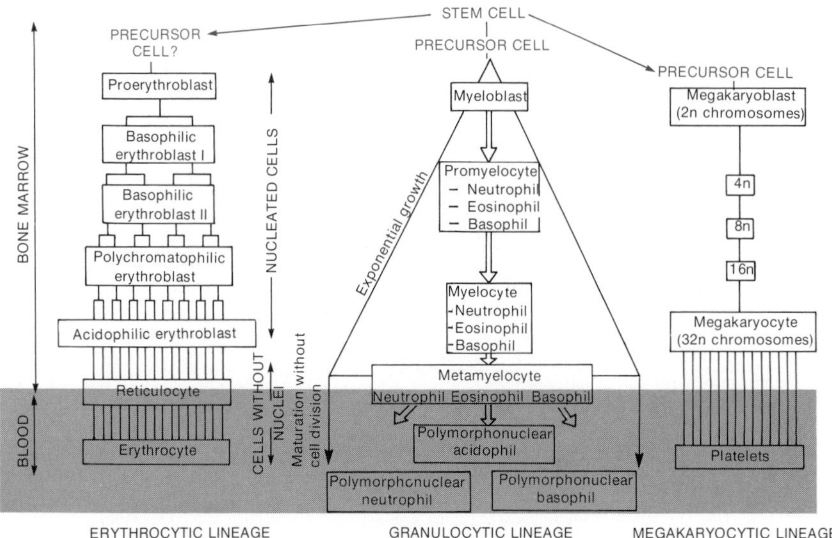

Figure 24. Maturation of blood cells.

need arises. They are self-perpetuating and guarantee the possibility of production throughout the life of an individual.

This cell pool responds to local influences (cellular interactions), which determines the CFU response in one way or another. Higher placed influences induced the CFU to enter the replication cycle, as needed, depending on the rate of release of these cells towards the pool of precursor cells.

Precursor Cell Compartment (ERC or ACU). Precursor cells are highly proliferative but the constituent cells are capable of only a limited number of divisions. This group is regulated by poietins.

Maturing Cell Compartment. These cells represent transitional stages between the stem cell compartment and the blood compartment. The maturing cells are the only ones that can be identified morphologically. At this level in the granulocytic cell line there is a final mode of regulation which permits the rapid mobilization of the granulocyte reserve and insures a supply in the event of urgent need.

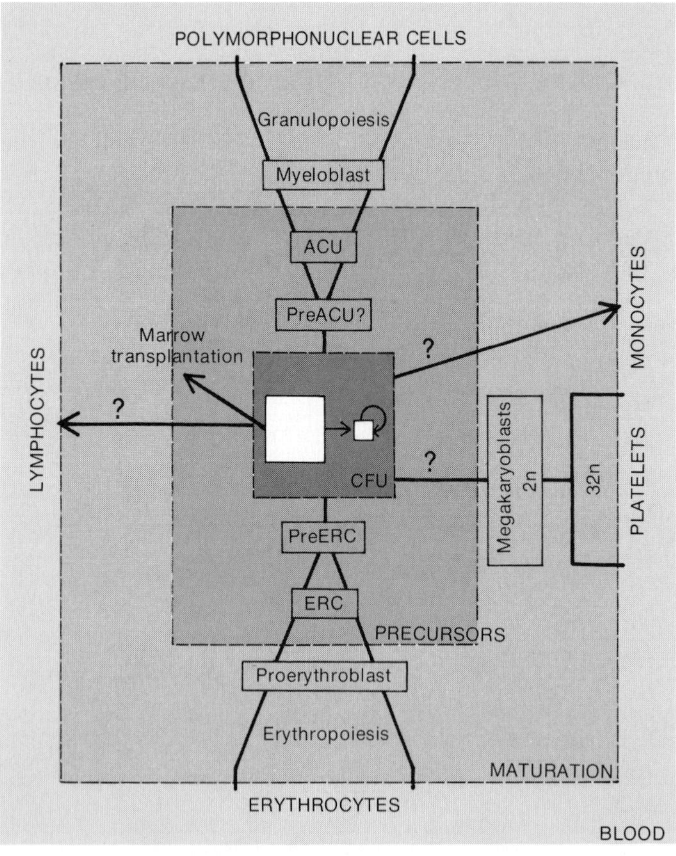

Figure 25. Hematopoietic compartments.

9

Skeletal Tissues

Bone and cartilage are connective tissue composed of cells, fibers, and ground substance. They differ from connective tissue proper by their solid consistency.

I. CARTILAGE TISSUE

I. Three Histological Types of Cartilage

Hyaline Cartilage. The voluminous cells (chondrocytes) possess a round central nucleus and a cytoplasm rich in glycogen and lipid droplets. They are located in small lacunae surrounded by an optically homogeneous

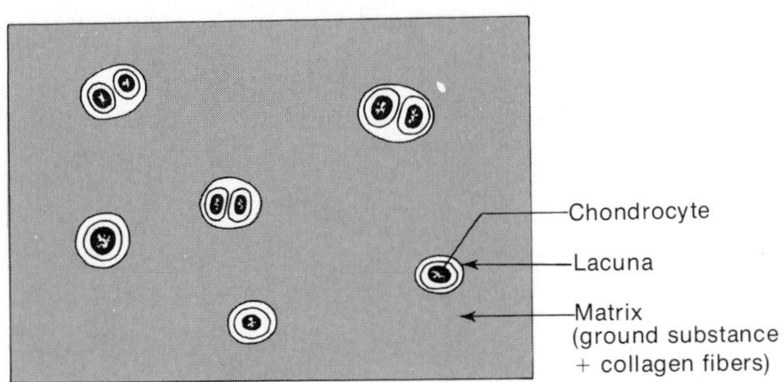

Figure 26. Hyaline cartilage as seen by light microscopy.

matrix made of mucopolysaccharide ground substance rich in chondroitin sulfate A and C. The ground substance contains fine collagenous fibrils forming large meshes visible only with the electron microscope.

Fibrocartilage. In comparison, fibrocartilage is richer in collagenous fibrils which, with the optical microscope, are visible as a closely woven network.

Elastic Cartilage. This type is characterized by the presence of numerous elastic fibers.

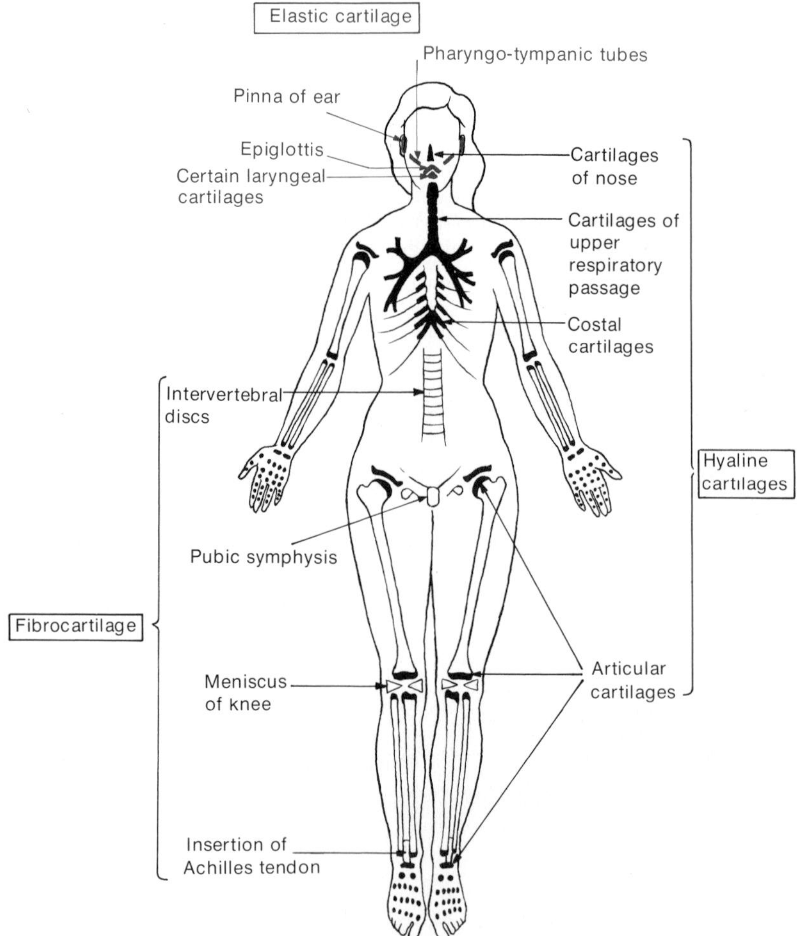

Figure 27. Distribution of the three types of cartilaginous tissue in the adult.

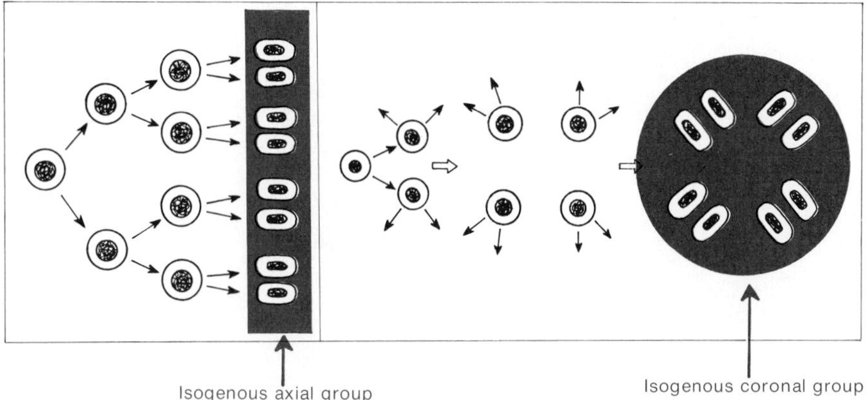

Figure 28. The two mechanisms of interstitial growth of the cartilage.

II. Histophysiology

The ground substance and collagenous fibers, as well as eventually the elastic fibers, are secreted by chondrocytes (or their precursors, the chondroblasts) in the same manner as connective tissue is laid down by fibroblasts.

Cartilaginous tissue does not contain blood vessels or lymphatic capillaries situated in the surrounding connective tissue (perichondrium).

Cartilage tissue growth occurs in two ways:

1. *Appositional growth,* by transformation of fibroblasts of the inner layer of the perichondrium into chondroblasts;

2. *Interstitial growth,* by mitoses of preexistent chondrocytes either linearly, producing isogenous axial cell groups, or circularly, giving rise to isogenous coronal groups.

II. BONE

A. ORGANIZATION OF BONE TISSUE

I. Constituting Elements of Bone Tissue

Cells

a. Osteoblasts. Osteoblasts are situated on the surface of growing bone tissue. They are roughly cuboidal in form, with elongated cytoplasmic

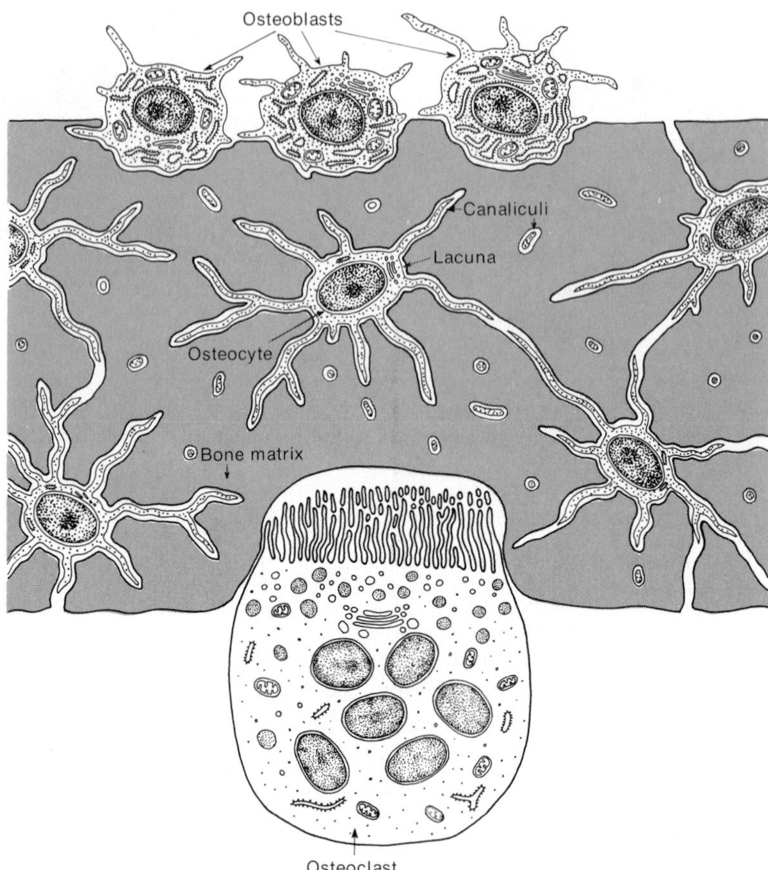

Figure 29. Diagram of bone tissue as seen by electron microscopy.

processes, and are rich in organelles, emphasizing their role in synthesis of proteins and glycoproteins.

b. Osteocytes. Osteocytes are osteoblasts completely embedded in mineralized ground substance. From the fusiform cell body, numerous thin cytoplasmic processes extend in all directions. Osteocytes reside in small lacunae from which canaliculi containing their cytoplasmic extensions branch out. Their organelles, of the same type as those of the osteoblasts, are less developed.

c. Osteoclasts. Osteoclasts are situated on the surface of bone tissue undergoing resorption, and are characterized by (1) their giant size, (2) multiple nuclei, (3) a brush border of irregular microvilli at the pole of the cell in contact with the bony matrix, (4) numerous cytoplasmic vesicles, (5) phagocytotic vacuoles, and (6) lysosomes, commonly grouped under the brush border.

Intercellular Matrix. This is composed of a mineralized organic substance (ground substance, collagenous fibers, and mineral salts).

a. Organic Matrix. Collagenous fibers are very numerous and present the usual structure. Ground substance, which is not abundant, contains mucopolysaccharides (especially chondroitin sulfate), glycoproteins, serum proteins, water, and electrolytes.

b. Mineral Salts. The hardness of bone depends on the mineralization of its organic matrix. This involves mainly hydroxyapatite crystals of calcium and phosphate, which are visible electron microscopically between the collagenous fibers. The ions Ca^{++} and PO_4^- on the surface of the crystals participate in rapid exchanges with the interstitial fluid, and thus with the bloodstream.

II. Formation and Resorption of Bone Tissue

During life, bone undergoes constant renewal owing to intricate processes of construction (formation of new bone tissue) and destruction processes (resorption of preexisting bone tissue). Thus, bone tissue carries out a metabolic role (release of mineral salts during destruction) and a supportive role (architectural adjustment to changes in mechanical conditions).

Formation of Bone Tissue

a. Formation of Pre-Osseous Substance by Osteoblasts. The osteoblasts (and, to a smaller extent, some osteocytes) synthesize and secrete glycoproteins and mucopolysaccharides, which later participate in the formation of the osseous ground substance. Tropocollagen molecules, released extracellularly, assemble into collagen fibers. From this organic matrix a pre-osseous, not yet mineralized, substance develops (osteoid tissue).

b. Mineralization. In the first step ("nucleation"), slightly soluble calcium phosphate is deposited between the collagenous fibers.

In step two ("crystallization"), hydroxyapatite crystals are constructed. The precise mechanism of bone tissue construction is very complex and not well understood.

Resorption of Bone Tissue. Two processes take place in the phenomenon of bone resorption.

a. Osteoclastic Resorption (Osteoclasia). A most important phenomenon is the resorption of bone tissue by osteoclasts. The osteoclasts excrete (by exocytosis): (1) H^+ ions, which dissolve mineral substances of bone tissue; (2) acid hydrolases (contained in the lysosomes), which depolymerize glucoproteins and mucopolysaccharides; and (3) collagenases, which attack the collagenous fibers. Residual fragments, remaining after acid and enzyme digestion, enter the osteoclast by endocytosis, where final "digestion" takes place. Parathyroid hormone stimulates the process of osteoclasia, through the intermediary action of adenyl cyclase and cyclic AMP of the osteoclasts.

b. Peri-osteocytic Resorption (Osteolysis). Some osteocytes have an activity that is more lytic than synthetic and, by unknown mechanisms, cause demineralization and lysis of surrounding bone tissue. This phenomenon starts with enlargement of the lacunae in which they are located.

B. BONE ORGANIZATION

I. Architecture of Bones

Whether long, short, or flat (see Fig. 30), all adult bones are made of lamellar bone tissue, either compact or spongy. Bone is surrounded by a layer of vascularized connective tissue (the periosteum), except where articular cartilages are found. All bones contain vessels and nerves.

Long Bones, Short Bones, and Flat Bones (see Fig. 30)

Compact Bone and Spongy Bone. Whether compact or spongy, adult bone tissue is always lamellated, which means that bone matrix is deposited in layers with parallel collagenous fibers, which alternate in direction with each successive layer. Between lamellae are located the lacunae containing the osteocytes.*

*However, primary bone tissue is not lamellar, which means that the matrix is not deposited in regular lamellae.

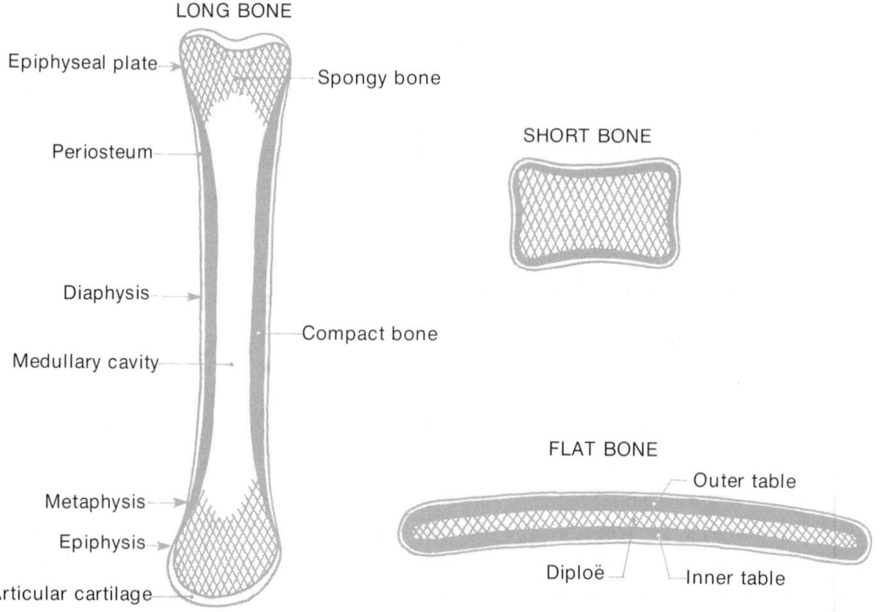

Figure 30. The three anatomical varieties of bone and the distribution of compact and spongy bone tissue.

a. Compact Bone Tissue. Compact bone (Fig. 31) is formed mainly of osteons or haversian systems, made of 4 to 20 cylindrical bony lamellae arranged concentrically around the osteonic canal. The canal contains blood capillaries and nonmyelinated nerve fibers covered by loose connective tissue. The osteocytes reside in the lacunae interposed between the lamellae. The haversian canals are connected with one another, with the medullary cavity, and with the bone surface by transverse or oblique canals (Volkmann's canals). This arrangement gives compact bone maximum strength. Between osteons are bone lamellae, remnants of old and partially resorbed osteons, making up the "interstitial systems." The diaphysis of long bones is bordered externally and internally by circumferential layers, the outer circumferential and inner circumferential lamellae.

b. Spongy Bone Tissue. Spongy bone is formed by a three-dimensional latticework of bony spicules or trabeculae which branch and anastomose, thus delimiting a labyrinth of intercommunicating spaces that are occupied by bone marrow (see Chapters 8 and 13) and vessels.

II. Formation and Growth of Bones

Whether they originate from an embryonic model of connective tissue or cartilage, all bones form as a result of differentiation of mesenchymal cells into osteoblasts, which secrete the organic matrix that later mineralizes.

Bones with a Connective Tissue Model (Intramembranous Ossification). These are found primarily in the small facial bones and in the flat bones of the skull. The formation and growth of these bones is direct and consists of a deposition of bone tissue inside connective tissue. Osteoblasts differentiate at ossification points which extend progressively. The nonlamellar bone tissue formed during primary ossification is replaced during secondary ossification by lamellar bone tissue, which is compact at the periphery and spongy in the center.

Bones with a Cartilage Model (Intracartilaginous Ossification). This process is concerned with long bones, short bones, and certain flat bones. The transformation of the embryonic cartilaginous model into the final adult bone ends only after puberty.

Primary Ossification of the Diaphysis. This results from two parallel yet separate processes, namely:

a. *At the periphery of the diaphysis,* intramembranous ossification starts at the inner layer of the perichondrium, which thus becomes the periosteum. It makes a loop and then a collar that becomes progressively larger and thicker (periosteal ossification);

b. *In the center of the diaphysis,* endochondral (intracartilaginous) ossification starts at an ossification point in the center of the diaphysis and

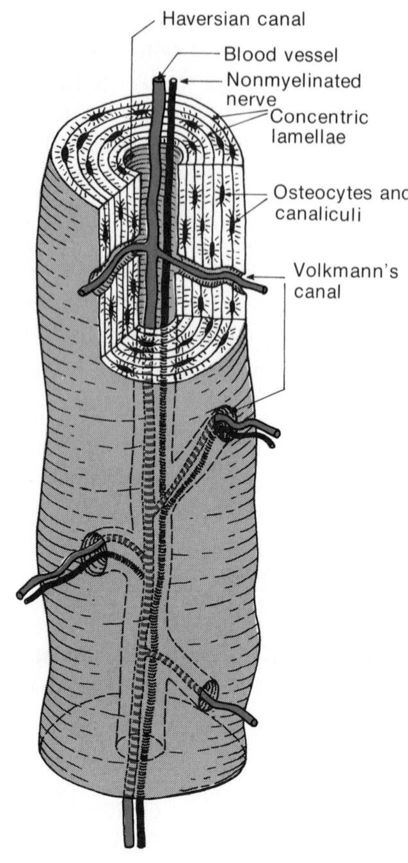

Figure 31. Three-dimensional diagram of an osteon (or haversian system).

progresses towards each of the two bone extremities. This ossification point is the site of several characteristic events:

1. Chondrocytes become hypertrophic; cytoplasm accumulates glycogen and becomes vacuolar; lacunae grow in proportion to the reduction in fine meshes of the cartilaginous organic matrix. These calcify by the deposition of hydroxyapatite crystals in the ground substance. Chondrocytes degenerate progressively and die, whereas the enlarged lacunae become confluent.

2. During this time, blood capillaries proliferate and enter into the open lacunae that became vacant owing to the death of the chondrocytes. These capillaries bring with them undifferentiated mesenchymal cells which differentiate into hematopoietic cells. Other mesenchymal cells, coming into contact with cartilage cells, differentiate into osteoblasts, which settle at the surface of the residues of the calcified cartilage matrix, and deposit a layer of bony tissue. Thus, osseous tissue progressively takes the place of cartilage tissue.

This zone of centrodiaphyseal intracartilaginous ossification is rapidly hollowed in its center by osteoclasts, which start shaping the future medullary cavity.

Primary Ossification of the Epiphysis. Primary ossification of the epiphysis is delayed until the primary ossification of the diaphysis is already well advanced. It begins with an intracartilaginous ossification, which progresses centrifugally from an ossification point in the center of the epiphysis. Intracartilaginous ossification does not extend to the whole epiphyseal sphere, but skips the articular cartilage.

Secondary Ossification. This follows the same general architectural plan of primary ossification, but completely modifies the structure of bone tissue. The nonlamellar bone tissue, whether derived from connective tissue or cartilage and whether diaphyseal or epiphyseal, is replaced by lamellar bone tissue.

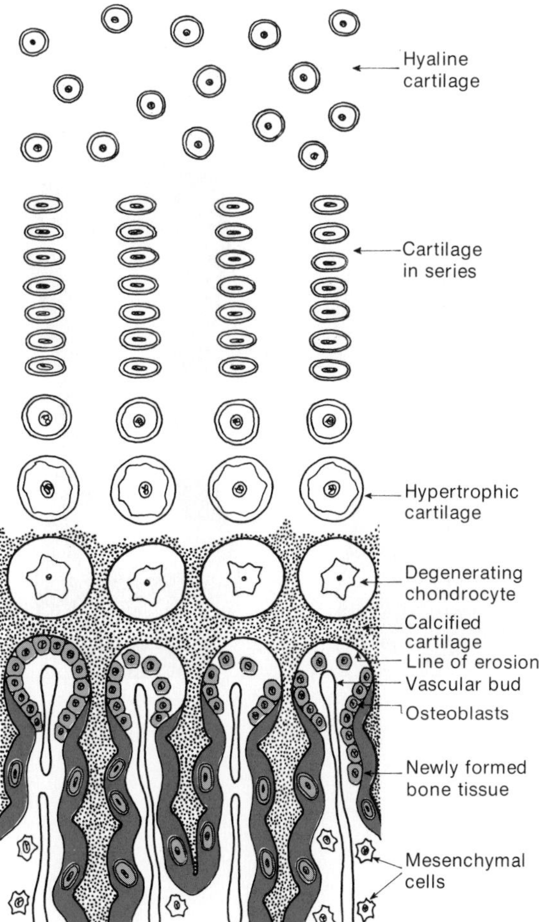

Figure 32. Endochondral ossification.

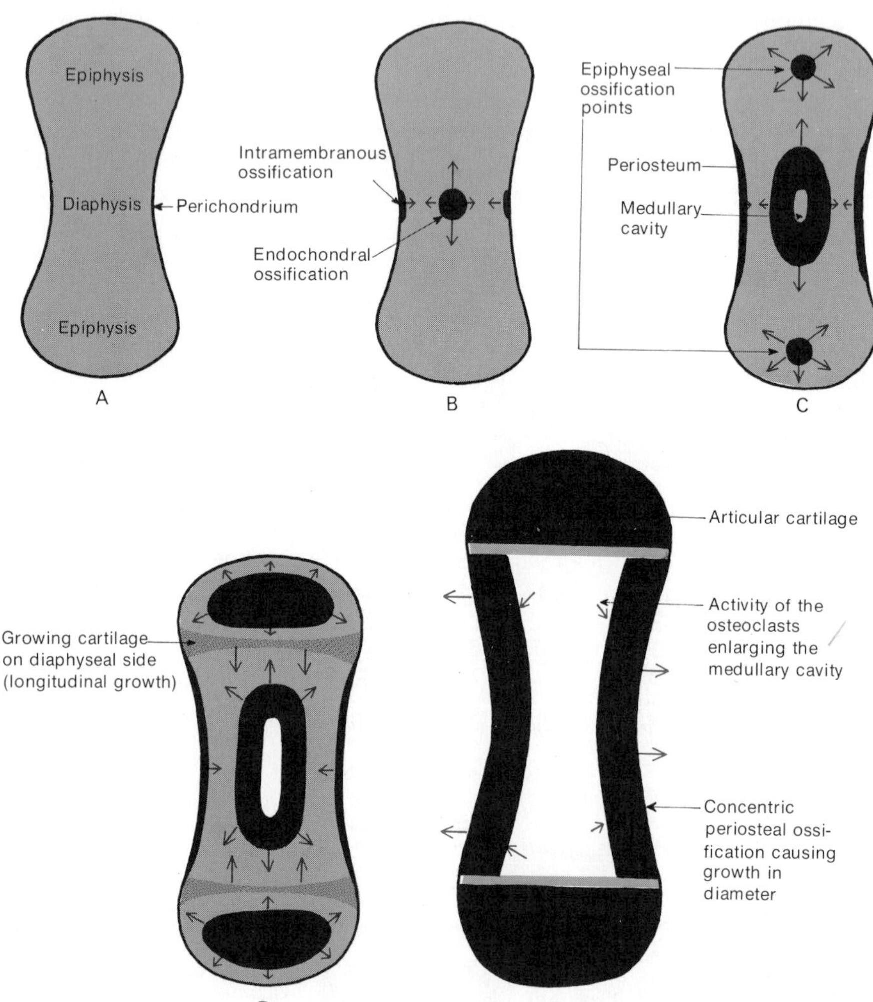

Figure 33. Formation and growth of bones.

Growth in Length. Such growth occurs by proliferation of the epiphyseal cartilage plate situated between the epiphysis and diaphysis. This plate is the site of multiple chondrocyte mitoses producing axial isogenous groups ("cartilage in series"). During growth according to this mechanism, they are replaced progressively by bone tissue because of the advancing intracartilaginous ossification from the center of the diaphysis. When all cartilage has been replaced by bone tissue, and when no more chondrocytes undergo division, growth in length is terminated, usually between the ages of 20 and 25.

Growth in Diameter. Growth in diameter occurs by successive apposition of new bone layers at the periphery as a result of activity of the periosteum ("periosteal ossification" of the intramembranous type). Simultaneously, osteoclast activity leads to the enlargement of the medullary cavity.

10

Muscle Tissue

Muscle cells, specialized to perform mechanical work (muscular contraction), are characterized by the presence of filamentous contractile proteinaceous material, the myofilaments. There are two types: thin filaments of actin, and thick filaments of myosin grouped to form myofibrils.

A. SMOOTH MUSCLE TISSUE

I. The Smooth Muscle Cell

The smooth muscle cell, which is fusiform and elongated, possesses: (1) a central nucleus; (2) a cytoplasm with two zones: one contains the vital organelles and caps the two poles of the nucleus; the other occupies the greater part of the cell and is packed with myofilaments; and (3) a plasma membrane covered by a basal lamina. Bundles of collagen fibers are inserted into the basal lamina. At certain points, the plasma membranes of two adjacent cells form "nexuses"—zones which permit the spread of excitation from one cell to another.

II. The Contractile Apparatus

Myofilaments are grouped into irregular fascicles (the myofibrils), which are disposed parallel to the long axis of the cell. With the electron microscope, small dense areas are seen on both the external and internal faces of the sarcolemma, which are insertion sites of the myofilaments.

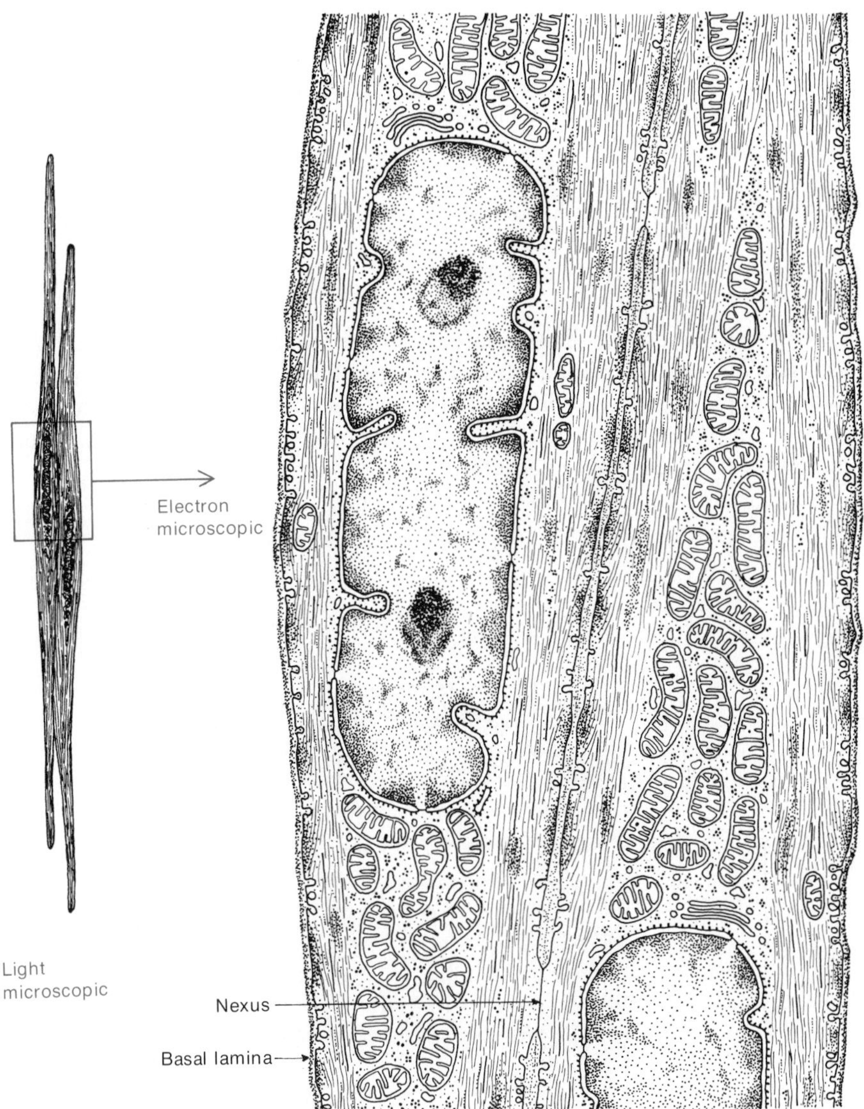

Figure 34. Smooth muscle cells. (From T. L. Lentz, 1971.)

Contraction of smooth muscle cells is involuntary, but may be spontaneous (myogenic contraction), or depend on the sympathetic and/or parasympathetic nervous system which innervates it (neurogenic contraction).

III. Organization

Smooth muscular cells occur either singly or in groups. In the latter case, a fine network of collagenous fibers provides the necessary cohesion.

B. STRIATED SKELETAL MUSCULAR TISSUE

I. The Striated Muscle Cell*

General Structure. The striated skeletal muscle cell, surrounded by a basal lamina, has the shape of an oblong cylinder, and possesses several hundred nuclei located peripherally against the sarcolemma. Its cytoplasm contains the usual cell organelles and numerous glycogen particles. There are, however, three main characteristics:

---

*Striated muscle cells are often (but improperly) called "striated muscle fibers."

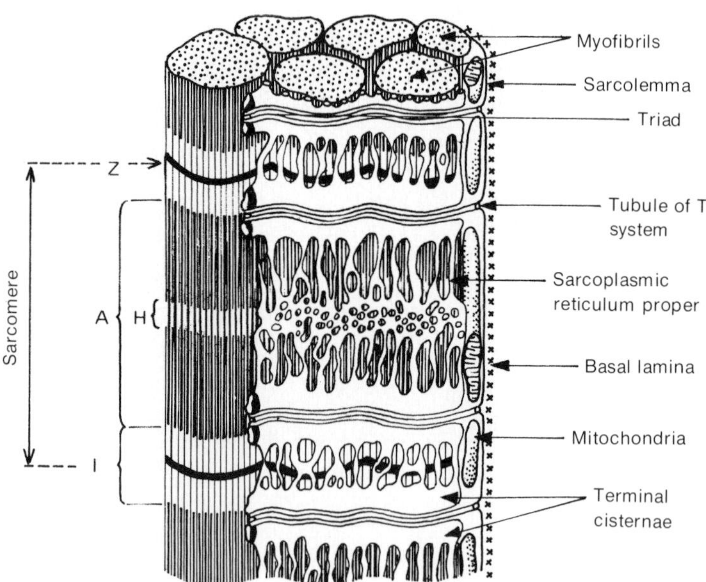

Figure 35. Organization of myofibrils and sarcoplasmic reticulum of skeletal striated muscle cells.

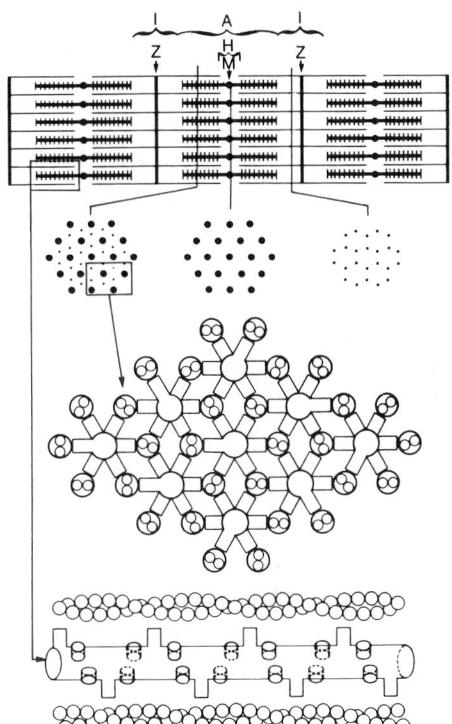

Figure 36. Diagram of the structure of a sarcomere as seen by electron microscopy. (After H. E. Huxley.)

a. Myofibrils. These are parallel cylinders lying in the longitudinal axis of the cell. They are made up of small repeating identical units called sarcomeres. Each sarcomere is made up of a fascicle of myofilaments oriented parallel to its long axis. The arrangement of the two kinds of myofilaments (actin and myosin) within the sarcomere forms the basis of the regions visualized as transverse striations of the myofibrils with the light microscope.

Myosin filaments are arranged in the middle of the sarcomere at the site of the A zone. In the H zone, myosin filaments are the only ones present. However, in the lateral parts of the A zone, the thin filaments and the thick filaments interdigitate. The thin filaments are arranged between the thick filaments in a regular hexagonal array with connecting bridges. At the level of the I zone, only thin filaments are present. At the Z line, the ends of the thin filaments of two adjacent sarcomeres interpenetrate over a short distance, having at this level a dual system of bridges between the thin filaments of each of the two sarcomeres.

b. Smooth Endoplasmic Reticulum. Smooth endoplasmic reticulum or *sarcoplasmic reticulum* is made up of a network of longitudinal canaliculi and anastomosing saccules, surrounding each myofibril and ending as terminal cisternae at the level of each junction between the A and I zones.

c. The T System. The *T system* is formed by a transverse system of canaliculi (tubular invaginations of the sarcolemma) surrounding the myofibrils at the junction between A and I zones. At that level, they form "triads" with the abutting terminal cisternae of the sarcoplasmic reticulum.

d. Abundant Mitochondria. The mitochondria, arranged linearly between myofibrils, supply the chemical energy (ATP) needed by the striated muscle cell to produce mechanical energy.

Muscular Contraction. Contraction of myofibrils results from modification of connecting bridges uniting actin and myosin filaments. As a result, the actin filaments slide between the myosin filaments, causing a shortening of the sarcomere ("contraction").

Structural modification of the bonds uniting myosin and actin is associated with a dephosphorylation of muscle ATP. This reaction depends on Ca^{++} ions present in a highly concentrated form in the cisternae of the sarcoplasmic reticulum. Depolarization of the plasma membrane depends on nerve impulses. Excitation is carried along the membranes of the T system, and is transferred to the sarcoplasmic reticulum through the triads. Depolarization of the triad membranes frees the necessary Ca^{++} and induces muscular contraction. Active reaccumulation of Ca^{++} within the sarcoplasmic reticulum stops ATP hydrolysis at the bridges and causes muscle relaxation.

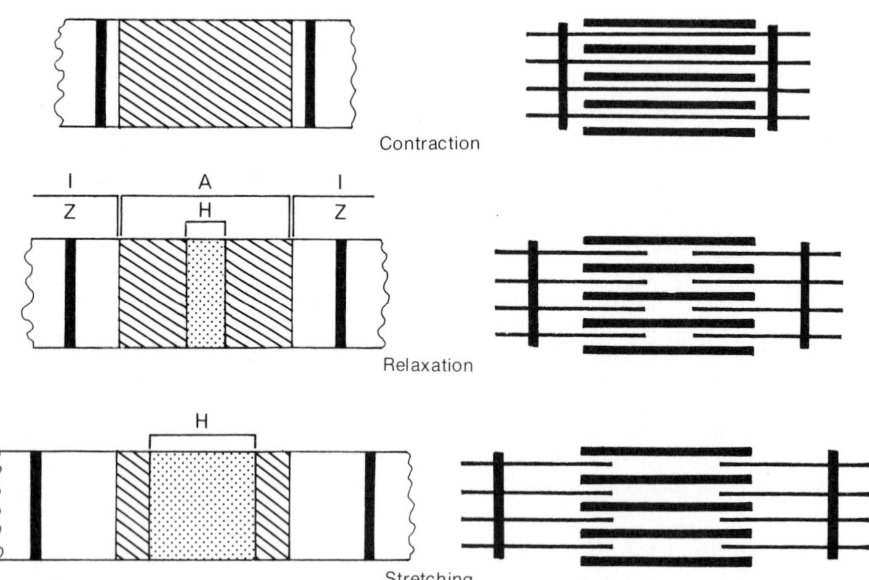

Figure 37. Mechanism of muscular contraction. *Left,* Changes in transverse striations of the sarcomere with different states of contraction. *Right,* Diagram illustrating the "sliding filament" hypothesis, showing interdigitation of actin and myosin filaments.

TABLE 13. Smooth Muscle Cells

Types		Histology	Location
Common Smooth Muscle Cells	Isolated	Connective tissue capsule or stroma of some entire organs (prostate, cavernous bodies, etc.)	
		Subcutaneous tissue (scrotum, areola and nipple of breast)	
		Lamina propria of the intestinal villi (Brücke's muscle)	
	Grouped	Tunicae (oriented layers)	Walls of hollow organs: blood and lymph vessels, digestive tract, and excretory ducts; tracheobronchial tree; urogenital ducts, uterus
		Individualized muscles	Arrector pili muscles of hairs, constrictor and dilator muscles of the iris, ciliary muscles
Specialized Smooth Muscle Cells	Ramose Cells	Star-shaped	Media of the large elastic arteries
	Myoepithelial Cells	Star-shaped molded on the acini	Exocrine glands of ectodermal origin (sudoriferous, salivary, mammary)
	Myoepithelioid	Dual muscular and secretory differentiation	Renin-secreting cells of the juxta-glomerular apparatus of the kidney

TABLE 14. The Two Principal Types of Skeletal Striated Muscle Fiber

Principal Characteristics	Fibers of Type I (Slow or "Red" Muscle)	Fibers of Type II (Fast or "White" Muscle)
Myoglobin	+++	+
Mitochondria	+++	+
Oxidative Enzymes	+++	+
ATPase (at the level of the myofibrils)	+	+++

Different Types of Striated Muscle Cells. Although all striated muscle cells have a propagating potential and undergo phasic contraction, it is possible to distinguish at least two types of cells ("red" and "white" muscle fibers; see Table 14). Frequently an intermediate type is distinguished.

In a given species the composition of muscle in terms of cells of type I and of type II is remarkably constant, and there is a correlation between types of striated muscle cells and contractile properties of the muscle.

A motor unit* is formed by muscle cells of the same type. The muscle cell type ("slow" or "fast") is determined by the nerve cell, which has a permanent influence on it. Muscle cells do not appear to have an inherent metabolic individuality, and take their contraction characteristics from the nerves supplying them.

II. Nerve-Muscle Coupling

Motor End-Plate. In normal muscle, muscle cells contain unique innervations. At a certain point on the plasmalemma, there is a special structure where the myoneural junction occurs (the motor end-plate).

At this level, the terminal ramifications of the axon are surrounded by Schwann cells only. Each axon arborization rests in a gutter carved in the surface of the muscular cell. The axon lies in this synaptic gutter directly on the plasmalemma of the muscle cell, from which it is separated only by the primary synaptic cleft. It contains mitochondria and synaptic vesicles, and is covered on the upper surface by a Schwann cell. In the synaptic gutter the sarcolemma is indented by multiple parallel invaginations, making up secondary synaptic clefts that constitute the subneural apparatus, which is very rich in cholinesterase.

---

*A motor unit is formed by a motor neuron and the striated muscle cells which depend on it.

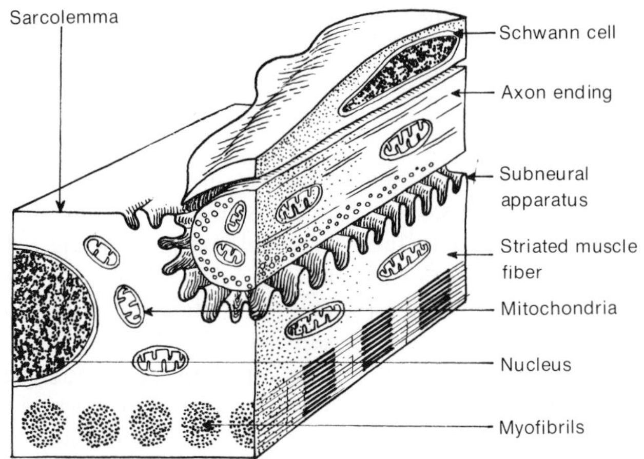

Figure 38. Schematic representation of the ultrastructure and three-dimensional aspect of a motor end-plate.

Transmission of Excitation to the Striated Muscle Cell. This is effected by the general mechanism of synaptic transmission (see Chapter 11, Nerve Tissue).

Depolarization of the presynaptic membrane, which transmits the nerve impulse, sets off the release of acetylcholine in the synaptic cleft from the synaptic vesicles. The acetylcholine modifies the cell's permeability to Na^+ and K^+ ions (acting on the membranes forming the subneural apparatus and causing their depolarization). The presence of excess amounts of cholinesterase ensures the instantaneous reversibility of transmission, so that the repolarized motor end-plate is available to transmit new impulses.

Trophic Influence of the Nerve on the Muscle. Within a motor unit, the dependency of the muscle cell on the motor neuron and its axon is demonstrated by cutting the axon. This induces muscle atrophy (denervation atrophy), which in turn causes degeneration of the motor endplates and subsequent myofibril modifications. Muscle atrophy is accompanied by characteristic metabolic and functional disturbances. There seems to be a regulating mechanism at the nerve level at which the modulating effect on the muscle cells acts independently of the processes that determine the workings of muscle contraction (nerve impulse).

III. Architecture of Skeletal Striated Muscles

Structure of a Striated Muscle. Skeletal muscle is composed of striated muscle cells grouped in fascicles held together by vascular connective tissue. An endomysium surrounds each cell, a perimysium surrounds the fascicles, and an epimysium encloses the muscle.

Skeletal muscles are inserted on tendons and through aponeuroses whose collagenous fibers arise at the extremities of each muscular cell. At this level, the sarcolemma shows more or less deep invaginations (muscle-tendon junctions).

Neuromuscular Spindles. These are encapsulated sensory receptors sensitive to degrees of tension and to the stretching speed of the muscle. They are arranged parallel to the extrafusal striated muscle cells and are composed of: (1) specialized striated muscle cells, called intrafusal cells; and (2) nerve fibers: the motor fibers (γ fibers) maintain the intrafusal cells at a certain degree of contraction. The sensitive fibers (especially Ia fibers), responding to stretching, are thus constantly kept just under their excitation threshold. When stretching occurs, the impulse from these nerve endings permits a feedback mechanism of control of muscular contraction strength (γ loop).

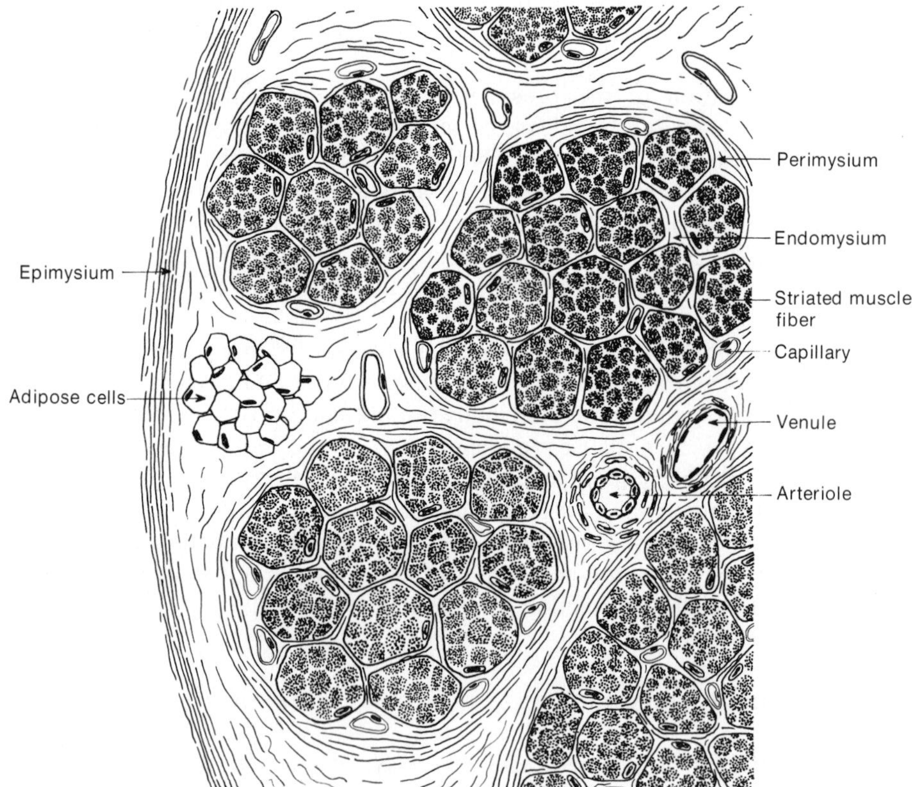

Figure 39. Light microscopic view of a skeletal striated muscle section.

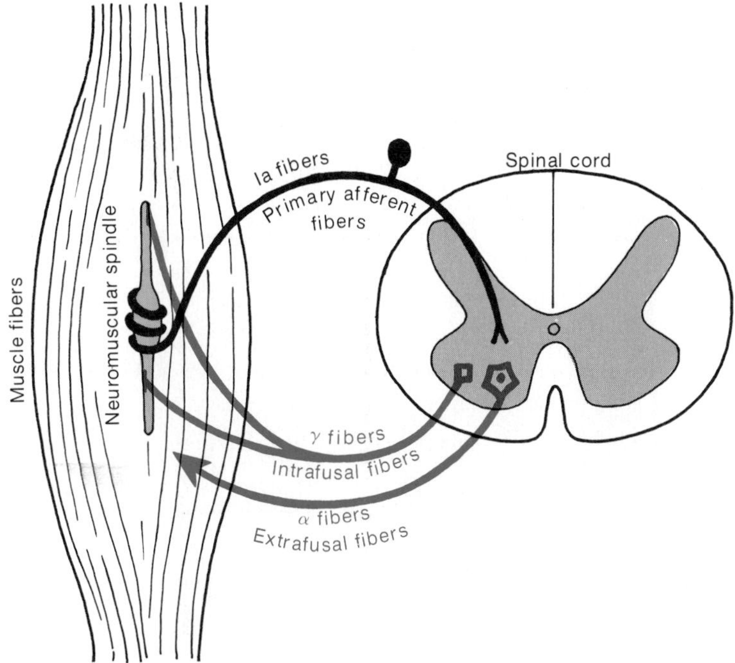

Figure 40. The γ chain of feedback control of the strength of muscle contraction.

C. CARDIAC MUSCLE TISSUE

Cardiac striated muscle tissue is characterized by its ability to contract rhythmically and harmoniously in a spontaneous manner.*

I. The Cardiac Striated Muscle Cell

This type of cell contains a single central nucleus and fascicles of parallel myofibrils with an elementary organization (sarcomere) similar to that of skeletal striated muscle cells. Mitochondria, glycogen, and sarcoplasmic reticulum also have similar morphological and functional importance. The cells have various shapes, but are mostly of a branched cylindrical type. Through these branches, they contact other cells to form a complex three-dimensional network.

---

*The heart is innervated by the autonomic nervous system. The rhythm of the heart pulsations is determined by the complex activity of the sinoatrial node and can be modified by sympathetic and parasympathetic influences.

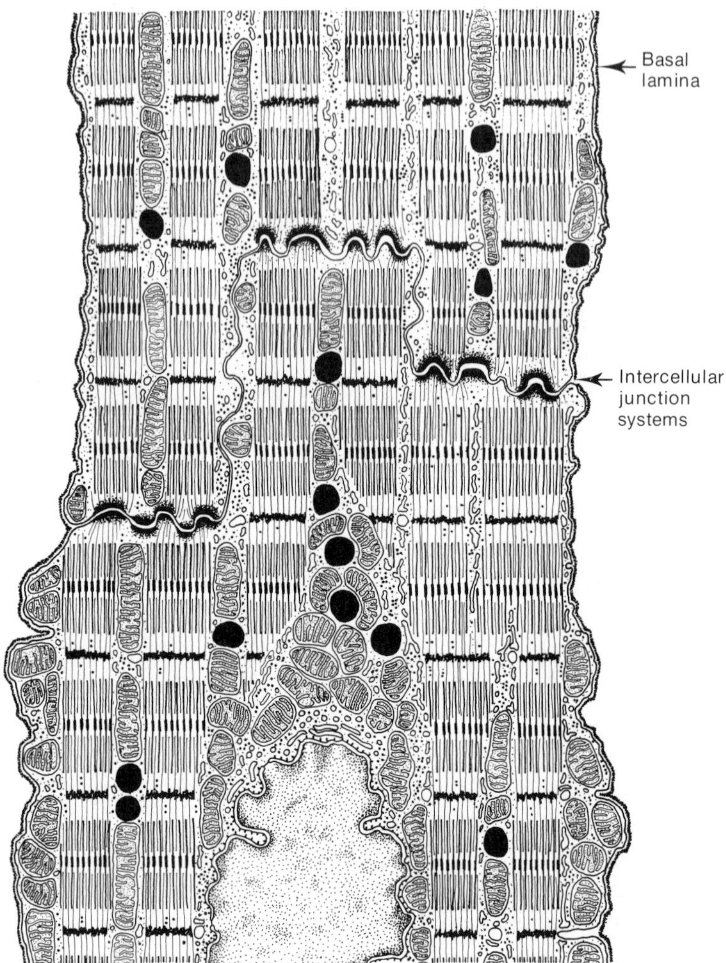

Figure 41. Cardiac muscle cells as seen by electron microscopy. (Modified after T. L. Lentz, 1971.)

The T system is not constant and is found in most cells of the ventricle and in some cells of the atrium, where it is located at the Z lines. Its function in cardiac muscle is not well known, since it does not appear to be essential for excitation-contraction coupling.

The sarcolemma has localized differentiations, which form areas of intercellular junctions (intercalated discs): macula adherens, zonula adherens, and/or zonula occludens. They are responsible for cell-to-cell transmission of tension developed by the myofibrils, and for the rapid cell-to-cell spread of excitation throughout the heart. Their nature and number determine the speed with which excitation is conducted and transmitted.

TABLE 15. Cardiac Striated Muscle Cells

<table>
<tr><th></th><th colspan="4">Cells Primarily Responsible for Intracardiac Conduction (Conduction System)</th><th colspan="3">Cells Primarily Responsible for Contractions of the Myocardium</th></tr>
<tr><td>CELLS</td><td colspan="3">Node Cells</td><td>Purkinje Cells</td><td colspan="2">Atrial Cells</td><td>Ventricular Cells</td></tr>
<tr><td rowspan="2">LOCATION</td><td rowspan="2">Sino-atrial node</td><td rowspan="2">Atrio-ventricular node</td><td colspan="2">Bundle of His</td><td colspan="2" rowspan="2">Atria</td><td rowspan="2">Ventricles</td></tr>
<tr><td>Trunk</td><td>Branches</td></tr>
<tr><td>SHAPE</td><td colspan="3">Oval, unbranched</td><td>Very large; branched, cylindrical</td><td colspan="2">Elliptical</td><td>Branched, cylindrical</td></tr>
<tr><td rowspan="2">MYOFIBRILS</td><td colspan="7">Identical organization in parallel fascicles formed by a succession of sarcomeres</td></tr>
<tr><td colspan="3">Scattered, scarce</td><td colspan="4">Occupy all of the cell except perinuclear region</td></tr>
<tr><td>MITOCHONDRIA</td><td colspan="3">Small, scarce</td><td colspan="4">Voluminous and numerous (especially in ventricular cells)</td></tr>
<tr><td>GLYCOGEN</td><td colspan="3">Absent or few</td><td>Large cytoplasmic areas separating the myofibrils</td><td colspan="3">Present between myofibrils and mitochondria</td></tr>
<tr><td>SARCOPLASMIC RETICULUM</td><td colspan="7">Very well developed</td></tr>
<tr><td>T SYSTEM</td><td colspan="5">Absent</td><td></td><td>Present with diads</td></tr>
<tr><td>JUNCTION SYSTEMS</td><td colspan="3">Rare; no specialized structures</td><td>Cells arranged in mosaics; specialized structures uniting lateral sides and extremities</td><td colspan="2">Specialized structures uniting lateral sides; oriented according to fiber axis</td><td>Specialized structures uniting ends of the cells; arranged perpendicularly to fiber axis</td></tr>
</table>

II. Heterogeneity of Cardiac Striated Muscle Tissue

Contraction, conduction, and transmission are the functions of all cardiac striated muscle cells. However, functional heterogeneity is expressed morphologically by: (1) presence of a T system, (2) form of the cell, and (3) type and organization of the junctional elements. Therefore, it is possible to distinguish:

a. Cells Whose Essential Function Is to Generate an Impulse. These cause myocardial cells (node cells) to contract, and then conduct this impulse (Purkinje cells); this is the cardiac conduction system.

b. Cells Whose Essential Function Is Contraction. Within this group there are great differences between atrial and ventricular muscle cells.

11

Nerve Tissue

I. NERVE TISSUE: SUPPORT OF THE NERVE IMPULSES

A. THE NEURON

The neuron (or nerve cell) receives information and produces a signal which it conducts and transmits. Each cell is unique, being neither equivalent to its neighbor nor interchangeable. Its uniqueness rests in its particular position within the nervous system and in its specific relationships to other neurons or to the periphery. Furthermore, the mature nerve cell does not divide, and the total stock of neurons is determined very early in an individual's life.

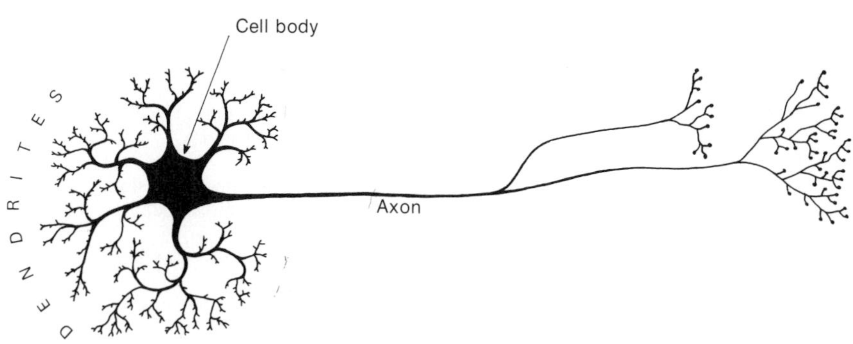

Figure 42. The neuron.

I. The Shape of the Neuron

The plasma membrane serves as the substratum for conduction of the nerve impulse. The nerve cell is made up of a cell body containing the nucleus and cytoplasmic processes.

Dendrites. Dendrites, usually short processes which conduct a nerve impulse towards the cell body, serve to extend the receptor zone of the cell. Their distribution within space determines the range of influences to which the neuron is submitted. Dendrites have irregular contours and may possess lateral synaptic protrusions (dendritic thorns), which increase greatly the receptor surface.

Axons. The axon is a single extension, but collaterals can branch out extensively. This structure originates on the cell body from a conical elevation (axon hillock), the region where the nervous impulse starts (after the depolarizing influences on the dendrites and cell soma have been summarized). The axon conducts this impulse from the cell body towards other neurons or effector cells. Its shape, like that of the dendrites, reflects its relationship to other structures, and therefore determines its location within the nervous system.

TABLE 16. Morphological Variations of Neurons

		Possible Variations	Characteristics
	CELL BODIES	Star-shaped Fusiform Conical Polyhedral Spherical	
	CELL BODIES	Pyramidal	Depending on size, can distinguish small, medium, large, and giant cells
DENDRITES	SPATIAL ORGANIZATION	Isodendritic	Branching in three dimensions
DENDRITES	SPATIAL ORGANIZATION	Allodendritic	Limited asymmetry
DENDRITES	SPATIAL ORGANIZATION	Idiodendritic	Specific organization
DENDRITES	ORGANIZATION WITH RESPECT TO THE CELL BODY	Unipolar	Only one extension (neuroblast)
DENDRITES	ORGANIZATION WITH RESPECT TO THE CELL BODY	Bipolar	One efferent and one afferent extension
AXON	ORGANIZATION WITH RESPECT TO THE CELL BODY	Pseudounipolar	Only one extension, branching off at a distance from cell body
AXON	ORGANIZATION WITH RESPECT TO THE CELL BODY	Multipolar	Multiple extensions
AXON	LENGTH	Long: Golgi Type I	Reaches regions away from the cell body
AXON	LENGTH	Short: Golgi Type II	Stays close to the cell body

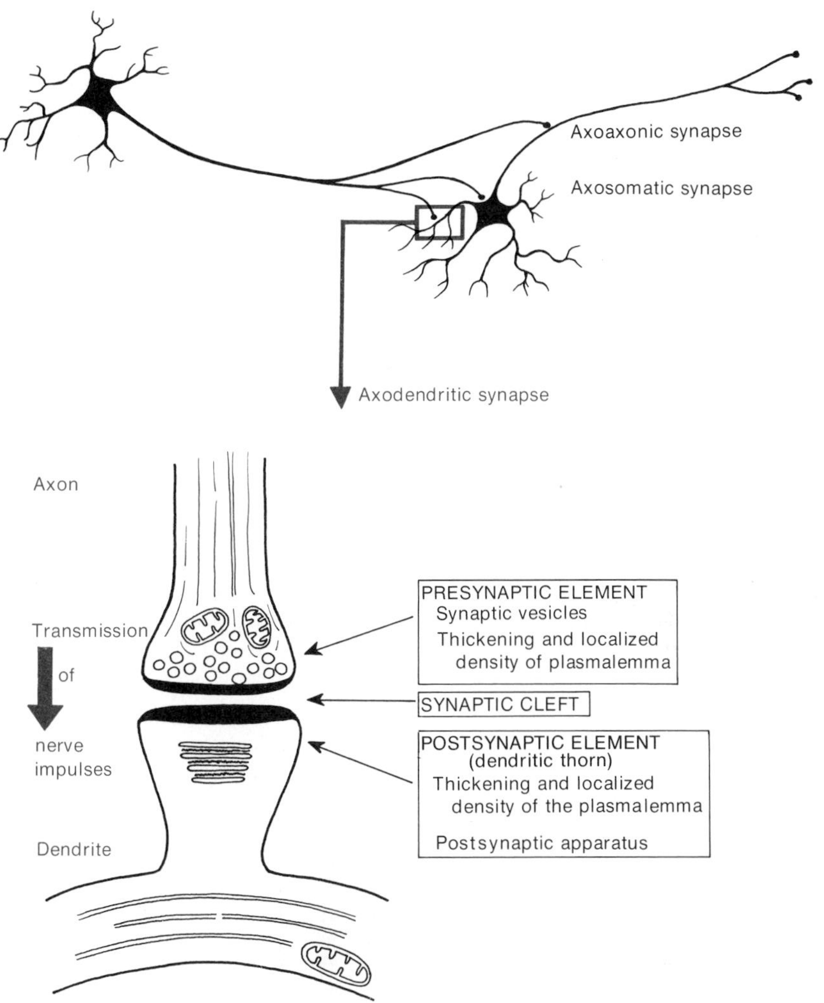

Figure 43. The synapses.

II. Synapses (Fig. 43)

At certain points on the neuron plasmalemma, there are differentiations where unidirectional cell-to-cell impulse transmissions occur (the synapses). There are no morphological features to predict the excitatory or inhibitory effect of the presynaptic elements on the postsynaptic element.

In humans, synapses transmit nerve impulses by a chemical mechanism. The synaptic vesicles represent transport and storage of neurotransmitters.

Each neurotransmitter has an exclusive character, making it possible to distinguish cholinergic, catecholaminergic, and serotoninergic synapses. When action potentials (nerve impulses) arrive at the presynaptic element, they initiate mobilization of synaptic vesicles towards the presynaptic membrane, and release of the neurotransmitter in the synaptic cleft. Action potentials, thus aroused, are propagated by the postsynaptic neurons. Once released, the transmitter is partially destroyed and partially reabsorbed by the presynaptic extremity. The membranous systems of the synaptic vesicles form the basis for storage and recapture.

B. MYELIN

Some axons are surrounded by a lamellar lipoprotein structure (the myelin sheath), which when examined with the electron microscope after fixation with osmic acid, appears as a spiral with a regular arrangement.

I. Myelinogenesis

The myelin sheath differentiates from the cell membrane of a satellite cell of the neuron. These cells sheathe the axon over a certain distance (interannular segment), so that the myelin sheath of an axon represents a sequence of identical myelin segments, separated by nodes of Ranvier.

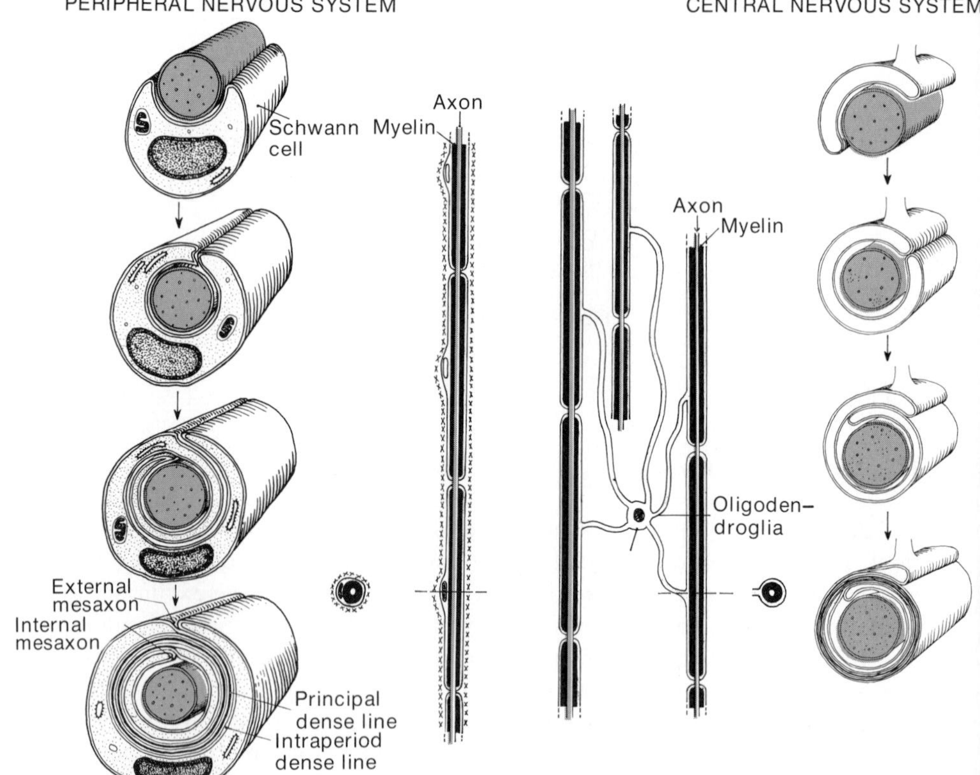

Figure 44. Myelin and myelinogenesis.

The formation of the myelin sheath starts with the invagination of the axon into the cytoplasm of the Schwann cell, eventually surrounding it completely and forming a mesaxon. The mesaxon in turn lengthens and forms a spiral around the axon. The cytoplasm, sandwiched between consecutive spirals of the mesaxon, later disappears when they fuse. Fusion of internal cell membrane layers forms the principal periodic dense line, and fusion of the external layers forms the intraperiodic dense line. The external and internal mesaxons persist over the whole longitudinal length of the spiral.

II. Myelin and Conduction Speed

One can distinguish between nonmyelinated and myelinated axons, observing in the latter great variations in the thickness of the myelin sheath. There is a relationship between axon diameter and the number of spirals, which determine this thickness and the length of the interannular segments.

The nodes of Ranvier, which are devoid of myelin, represent a zone of weak electric resistance and a site where local currents pass, controlling the nerve conduction along the axon. In myelinated fibers, the saltatory (skipping) progression of the action potential results from the discontinuous structure of the fiber sheath.

The thicker the myelin sheath, the faster the speed of conduction. This relationship is the only physiological fact that can be linked to morphology, since the designation of myelinated or nonmyelinated gives no clue to functional significance.

C. INTERRELATIONSHIP OF NEURONS

The neuron is the fundamental constituent of the nervous tissue, but it receives its major significance from the synapses in which it participates. The study of morphological relations between nerve cells (by silver impregnation techniques) reveals that the neuronal apparatus is organized throughout the whole nervous system in such a way as to form the basis for its functional capacities. Indeed, there are, within nervous tissue, *neuronal chains* composed of neurons with the same synaptic relationships (i.e., serving the same dendritic or axonal areas, and contributing to the same functions). The properties of these neuronal chains depend closely on the morphology of their constituting elements. The degree of myelination of the axon and the number of synapses from the starting point of an impulse to its terminus determine the speed of conduction and its precision, each new synapse representing a modifying integration of the original signal.

Immunofluorescent studies of chemical transmitters have recently shown that the type of chemical synapse that occurs in a given situation is not a matter of chance. Rather, certain nervous structures and tracts have a specific mode of synaptic transmission (nigrostriatal inhibitory dopaminergic tract, for example).

II. NERVE TISSUE: METABOLIC ORGANIZATION

A. THE NEURON

I. The Cell Body

The cell body has much of the metabolic machinery of the neuron, containing the nucleus and the endoplasmic reticulum. The latter is highly developed. The Golgi complex is very important, and its enzymatic activities are very diversified. All are indicative of the occurrence of significant protein synthesis. Fully one third of the protein content is renewed daily. The greater part of this protein production serves to maintain or to renew the cytoplasm and its organelles.

Some cells show particular signs which are linked to special functions: i.e., neurons with melanin from the substantia nigra (neurosensory cells).

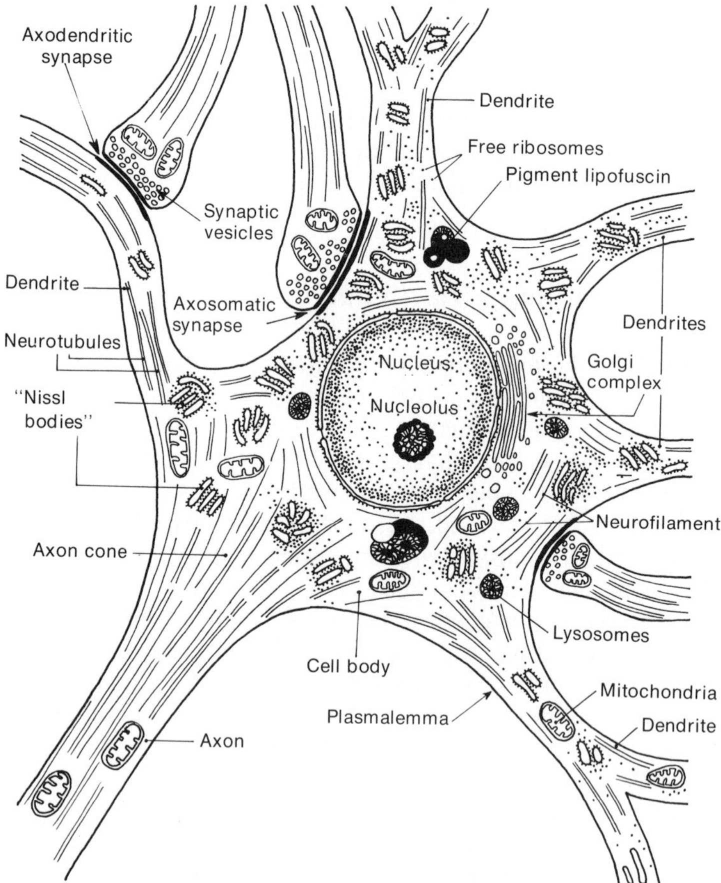

Figure 45. Schematic ultrastructure of a neuron.

TABLE 17. Distribution of Principal Organelles of the Neuron

	Dendrites	Cell Body	Axon		
			Cone	*Axon*	*Ending*
Nucleus		Spherical; often voluminous; pale, with big nucleolus			
Golgi Complex		Very well developed			
Endoplasmic Reticulum	Masses of flattened saccules of rough ER and of free ribosomes (Nissl body)		Progressive disappearance of ribosomes		
Neurotubules and Neurofilaments	Parallel fascicles of microtubules	Numerous, scattered and/or grouped	Microtubules		
				Parallel fascicles of micro-filaments	
	Identical to microtubules and filaments found in other cells; correspond to neurofibrils of light microscopy				
Mitochondria	Number increases as distance from cell body increases	Dispersed			Sometimes
Lysosomes	Some	Numerous	Some		
Lipofuscin	Sometimes	Abundant in the aged			
Synaptic Vesicles					Abundant

II. The Processes

Dendrites are processes of the cell body.

The *axon* is devoid of ribosomes, an aspect that is most manifest where the axon hillock joins the cell body. The axon is purely a conduction element and its components (proteins and enzymes) are synthesized in the cell body and brought peripherally to the extremity of the axon. The mechanism of this axonal flux is unknown, but apparently neurofilaments and neurotubules could play a role.

The axon is completely dependent on the cell body. If cut or injured, the distal extremity as well as its myelin sheath degenerates (wallerian degeneration). However, its proximal end has the capacity to regenerate. These phenomena are accompanied by an increased synthesis of RNA within the cell body. This is morphologically demonstrated by the occurrence of chromatolysis within the cell body.

B. NERVE TISSUE

Compared to the compact organization of the central nervous system, the peripheral nervous system is widely dispersed.

I. Central Nervous System

Constituting Elements. The central nervous system is composed chiefly of nerve cells, glial cells, and blood capillaries.

Glial Cells. These have processes intertwined with those of nerve cells. Several types are distinguished.

Astrocytes, which have processes extending in all directions, form structural support and insulate receptor surfaces of neurons (selectivity of impulse).

Oligodendrocytes are responsible for the formation of myelin sheaths in the central nervous system. One oligodendroglial cell can provide myelin for several axons.

Ependymocytes border the ventricular cavities.

Microglial cells do not seem to have a true neural individuality, but may be macrophages of the nervous system. They seem to originate mainly in the blood (monocytes) but some could spring from undifferentiated glial cells.

Spatial Organization

a. Gray Matter.* Gray matter corresponds to regions where interneuronal junctions (synapses) occur; at this level information is integrated

---

*The gray matter covers the surface of the cerebrum and cerebellum hemispheres (cortex) and also forms deep masses (gray central nuclei, gray axis of spinal cord).

TABLE 18. Glial Cells

	MACROGLIA			MICROGLIA
	Astrocyte		*Oligodendrocytes*	
	Protoplasmic	Fibrous		
Embryonic Origin	Ectodermal		Ectodermal	Mesodermal cells of the pia mater
Distinguishing Features	Large nucleus, abundant granular cytoplasm; numerous thick processes	Long, thin, smooth branched expansions	Smaller than astrocytes; smaller nuclei; few, slender processes with few branches	Smallest nuclei of all glial cells, which stain deeply; scant cytoplasm; few extensions twisted in various ways
Location	Many processes attached to blood vessels and to pia mater by expanded pedicles	Also attached to blood vessels	Relate intimately to nerve fibers in central nervous system	Scattered everywhere throughout the brain and spinal cord
	Chiefly in gray matter	Chiefly in white matter	In gray matter, principal type of satellite cell	
Role	Structural support; insulator of receptor surfaces; metabolic role (nutritional)		Form myelin in central nervous system; metabolic role?	Phagocytosis; great variety of forms with active migration
	Essential role in communications in the nervous system			

and the neuronal signals are produced. Thus gray matter comprises the grouping of the cell bodies and their processes, along with glial cells and capillaries, following a spatial (architectonic) organization inherent to each region. These elements, which constitute the neuropil, leave a space of 200 to 250 Å between their cell membranes, representing the extracellular compartment of the gray matter. The volume of this extracellular compartment is large, considering the contact surfaces between their countless processes. It represents 20 to 30 per cent of the total tissue volume and plays a fundamental role. Indeed, neurons have no direct contact with capillaries, and exchanges with blood are effected by the action of astrocytes or by diffusion within the extracellular space.

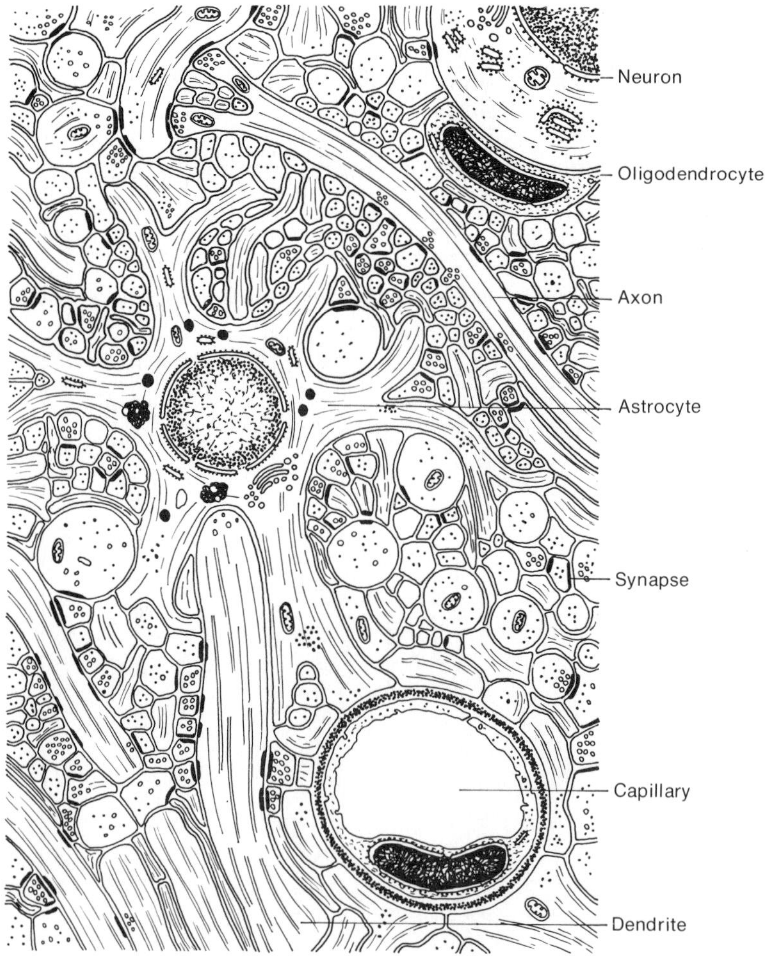

Figure 46. Diagram of gray matter as seen by electron microscopy.

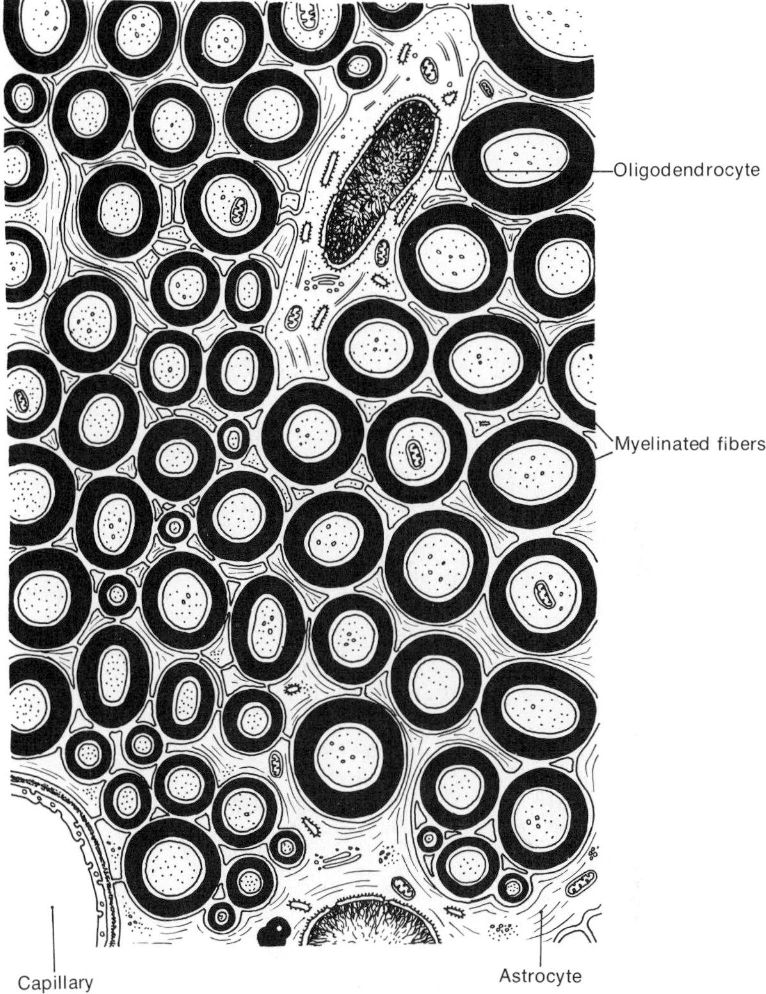

Figure 47. Diagram of white matter as seen by electron microscopy.

b. White Matter. Here the elements are also in contact but have little extracellular space. The predominant feature is the grouping of myelinated axons in fascicles. The glial cells are grouped among the axons, or elongated in the direction of their longitudinal axes. There are few capillaries. White matter is mainly conductive and its organization, which is linked to its lesser metabolic activity, differs greatly from that of gray matter.

Relationships of Nerve Tissue with the Other Components of the Central Nervous System. There exists, within the central nervous system, both a vascular and a fluid compartment (cerebrospinal fluid) with which the nerve tissue makes metabolic exchanges. Where possible, the structures in ques-

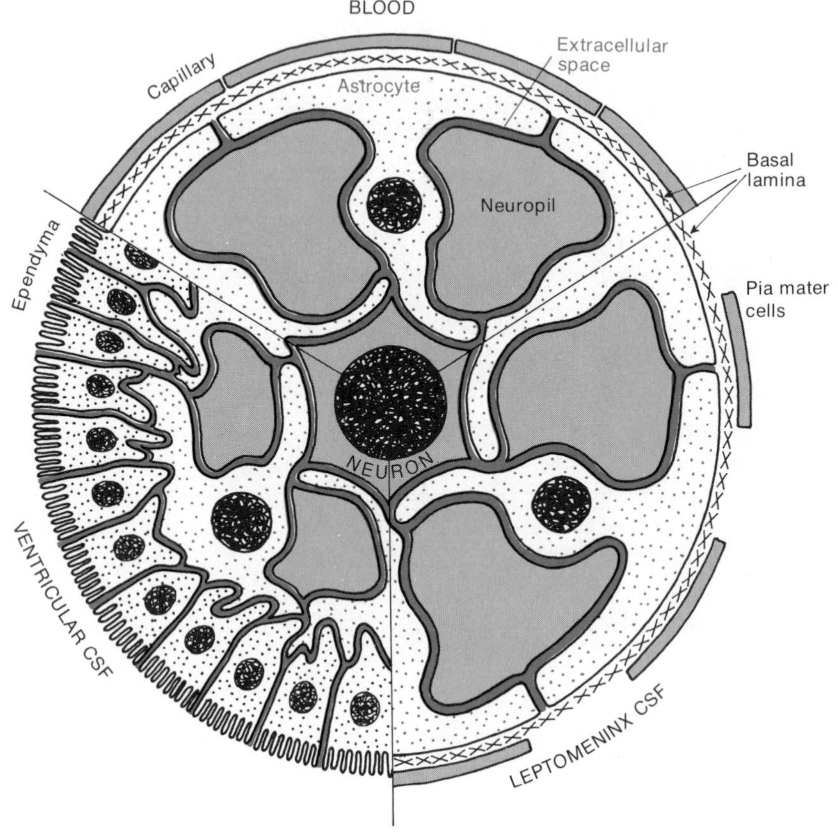

Figure 48. Diagram of the relationship between nerve tissue, blood, and cerebrospinal fluid.

tion are selective in these exchanges, a fact that forms the basis of the theory of barriers.

a. Blood-Brain Barrier. Exchanges between blood and nerve tissue, at least for large molecules such as peroxidase, depend on characteristics of the capillary endothelium (zonula occludens) and not on special relations between them and the vascular pedicles of the astrocytes.

b. Cerebrospinal Fluid (CSF)-Brain Barrier. Nerve tissue is in close contact with the CSF; the continuous layer of marginal astrocytes is separated from the CSF contained in the meshes of leptomeninges only by the basal lamina that borders them at the outside. In addition, the ependymal cells form a continuous cover. Their processes intermingle with those of the subependymal astrocytes. The ependyma barely hinders the passage of fluids and of large molecules between the ventricular system and the extracellular spaces of nervous tissue.

c. Blood-CSF Barrier. At certain points the ependymal epithelium undergoes a differentiation. Attached to a basal lamina and enclosing a vascular connective stroma, it forms the choroid plexuses. These produce CSF by active secretion (active transport of Na^+ and Cl^- through the choroidal epithelium).

II. Peripheral Nervous System

Constituents. The peripheral nervous system is made up of nerve cells, blood capillaries, and Schwann cells. These elements are enveloped by connective tissue, which is nonexistent in the central nervous system.

The Schwann cell is covered on the outside by a basal lamina. It is characterized and defined by the fact that it encloses: either (1) several

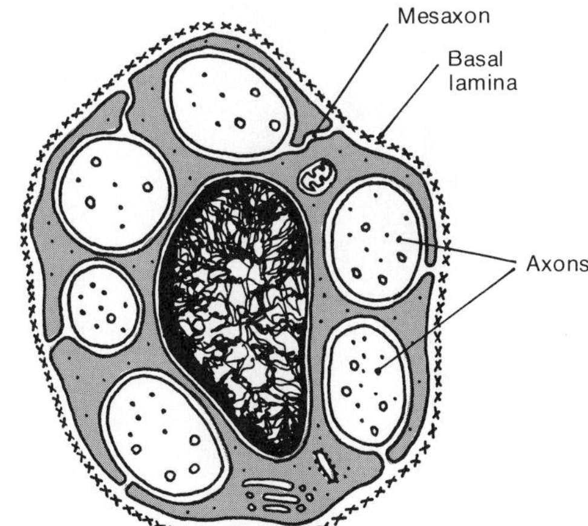

Figure 49. Cross-section of an unmyelinated nerve fiber.

axons, which invaginate in depressions of its cell membrane (unmyelinated nerve fiber)* or (2) a single axon, for which it forms the myelin sheath (myelinated nerve fiber).

Organization of the Peripheral Nervous System

a. Ganglia. Ganglia are masses of neuronal cell bodies surrounded by capsule cells (similar to Schwann cells). The sensory cranial and spinal ganglia do not contain synapses, but synapses do exist in the ganglia of the sympathetic and parasympathetic systems.

b. Peripheral Nerves. These are made up of peripheral nerve fibers grouped in fascicles. There is great variation from one nerve to the other, in the proportion of unmyelinated versus myelinated fibers, and in the thickness of myelin sheaths. As in the central nervous system, the peripheral nerve fibers located at the outside of these fascicles are "protected" by perineurium and capillary endothelium, which form barriers to moderate fluid exchange.

---

*Peripheral nerve fiber = neurite (axon or dendrite) + Schwann cell complement.

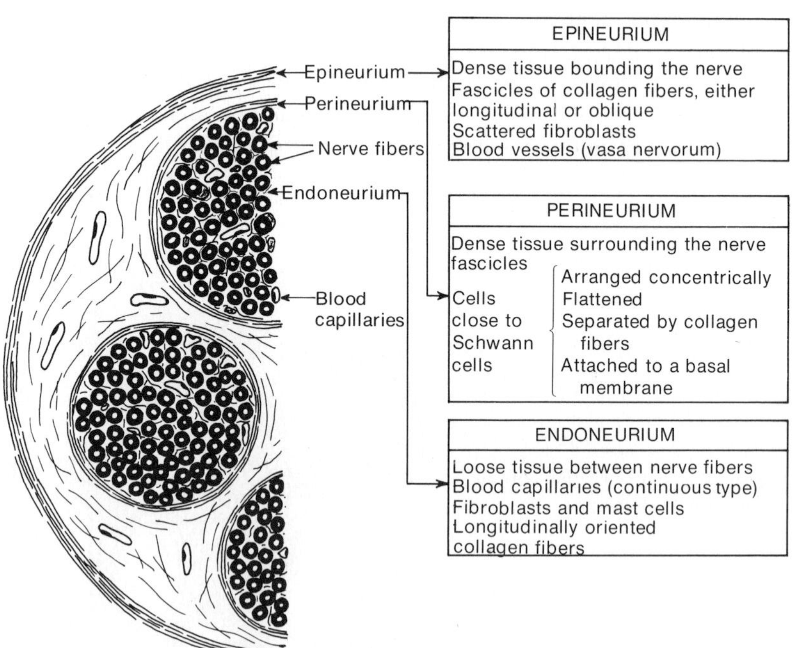

Figure 50. Cross-section of a peripheral nerve.

TABLE 19. Sensory Receptors

Category	Name or Type	Location	Receptor Function
Free Nerve Endings	Naked nerve fibers	Cornea	Touch
	Naked branches of the neuron	Each branch covers large area, as in the cornea	Pain
	Naked nerve fibers	Skin, most connective tissues	Pain
	Basket-like arrangement of nerve fibers	Base of hairs	Movement
	Merkel's discs: expanded discs on terminal twigs in stratified squamous epithelium	Border of tongue and other sensitive epithelia	Touch
Encapsulated Receptors	Corpuscle of Vater-Pacini	Subcutaneous tissue, joints, tendons, interosseous membranes, perimysium, mucous membranes, serous membranes, pancreas, heart, dermis, cornea	Deep pressure and vibration
	Genital corpuscles	Skin of external genitalia, skin of mammary gland	Pressure
	Meissner's corpuscles	External genitalia, nipples, lips, connective tissue papillae, palmar surface of hands, fingers, mucous membranes of eyelids	Touch
	Corpuscles of Ruffini	Deep in skin or even subcutaneous tissue, particularly plantar surfaces of foot	Warmth
	Krause's end-bulb	Dermis of conjunctiva, mucosa of tongue, mucosa of external genitalia	Cold
	Neuromuscular spindles	Found with striated muscle cells	Stretch reflex
	Neuromuscular organ	Junctions of muscles and tendons, aponeuroses of muscles	Tension

c. Nerve Endings

AFFERENT NERVE ENDINGS. These are receptors able to transform mechanical, chemical, thermal, and electrical stimulation into an afferent message. The fundamental and essential structural element is the termination of their peripheral processes in spinal or cranial ganglia.

The morphological variety of sensory endings has no clear physiological correlation. Some receptors, like the neuromuscular spindle, have a clearly defined role, but most cannot fit any special category of sensory modality.

EFFERENT ENDINGS. The best known variety is the neuromuscular junction, or motor end-plate. The efferent endings at the level of smooth muscles and glands are free endings.

PART THREE

ORGANS AND SYSTEMS

12

Cardiovascular System

A. BLOOD CAPILLARIES

Blood capillaries are sites of exchanges between blood and tissues.

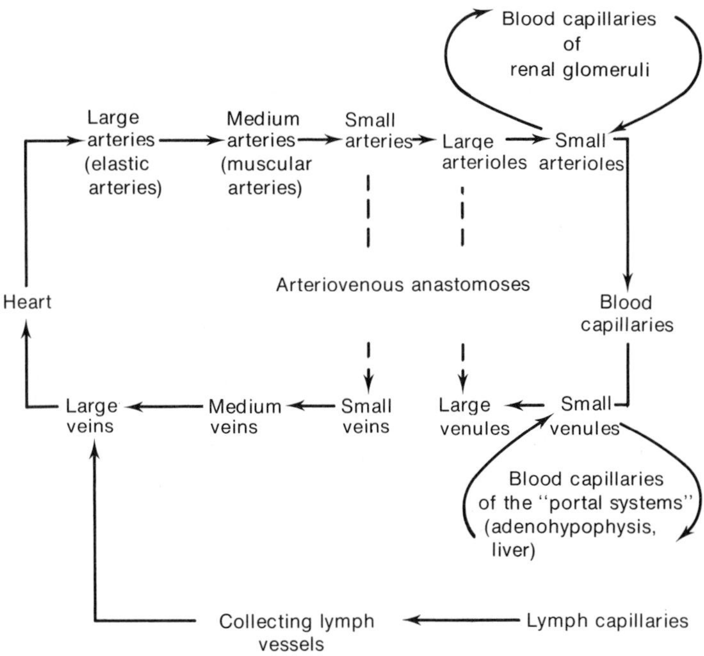

Figure 51. Diagram of the principal elements of the cardiovascular system.

I. Continuous Capillaries

Small caliber continuous capillaries are the most widespread in the organism. Their walls are made of a layer of connected squamous endothelial cells, surrounded by a continuous basal lamina that overlaps at certain points to enclose another cell, called the pericyte, which molds itself to the endothelium.

Exchanges between blood and tissues occur either through simple dif-

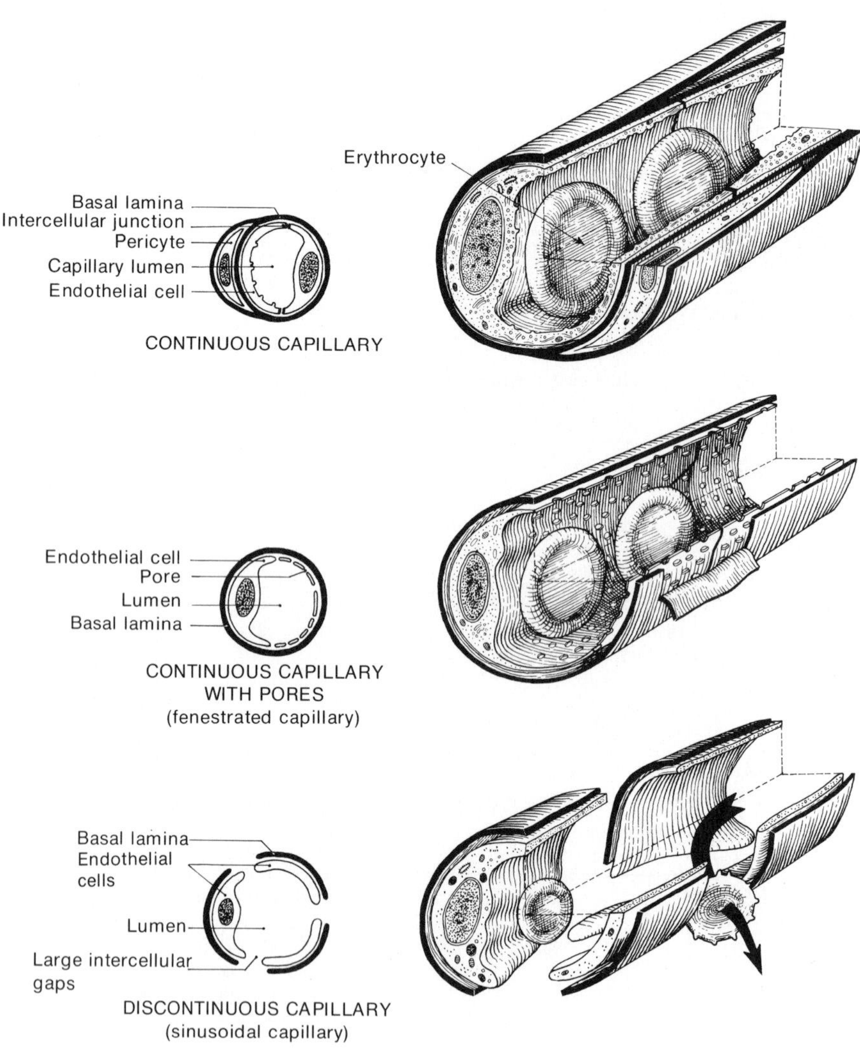

Figure 52. Blood capillaries. *Left,* Cross sections as seen by electron microscopy. *Right,* Three-dimensional reconstructions. (After J. Poirier and J. Nguyen H. Anh, La Presse Medicale, *75*:28, 1967.)

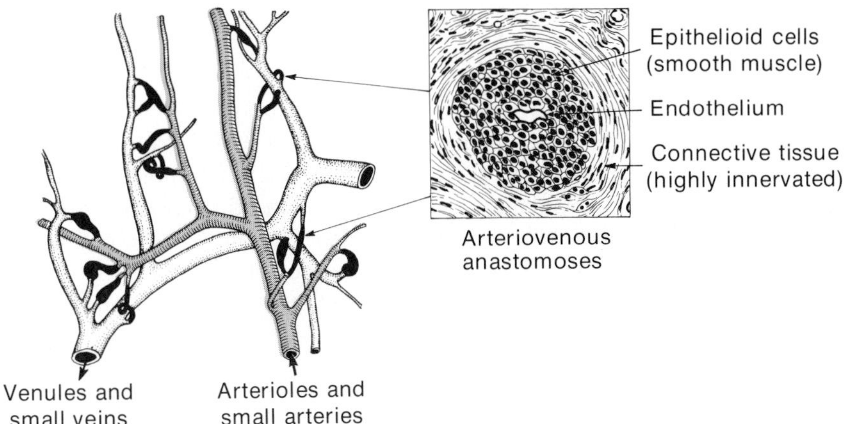

Figure 53. Arteriovenous anastomoses. (Redrawn after M. Clara, 1956.)

fusion (for O_2, CO_2), through intercellular junctions of the endothelium (for water, electrolytes, small molecules), or through the endothelial cell itself by way of very numerous micropinocytotic vesicles contained therein (for large molecules). Capillaries are passive, noncontractile tubes. Blood flow is regulated by precapillary sphincters at the origin of capillaries (a group of smooth muscle cells which are highly innervated) and by smooth muscle contraction of "junctional capillaries," which can short-circuit the true capillary bed.

The arteriovenous anastomoses also take part in the regulation of the capillary blood flow, since by opening, they can short-circuit the network of arterioles, junctional capillaries, true capillaries, and venules by establishing a direct arteriovenous "shunt." These structures, which exist in great numbers in the nail bed and the skin of the palms of hands and fingers, and on the soles of feet and toes, are formed by a sinuous canal connecting an arteriole to a venule.

In some organs, where there is extensive liquid exchange (endocrine glands, renal glomerulus, choroid plexus, and so forth), the cytoplasm of endothelial cells is pierced by multiple pores which are sometimes obstructed by a fine membrane ("fenestrated capillaries").

In the central nervous system, capillaries are enclosed entirely by the cytoplasmic processes of astrocytes instead of being surrounded, as in all other organs, by a pericapillary connective tissue space. Furthermore, instead of having endothelial cells joined by simple maculae occludentes, they are connected by zonulae occludentes that restrict the passage of certain substances ("blood-brain barrier").

Blood capillaries of erectile tissue are characterized by an irregular lumen, being either flattened or very dilated, according to physiological state (flaccidity or erection).

II. Sinusoidal Capillaries (or discontinuous capillaries)

These differ greatly from the preceding and exist only in the spleen, bone marrow, and liver. They form an integral part of the macrophage system. Indeed, their walls, which are discontinuous, are composed of macrophages ("bordering macrophages") that are separated from each other by large interstices through which certain formed elements of the blood pass (i.e., blood corpuscles). The basal lamina is either discontinuous or absent. Pericytes are also lacking. However, the capillaries are enclosed by a discontinuous feltwork of reticular fibers.

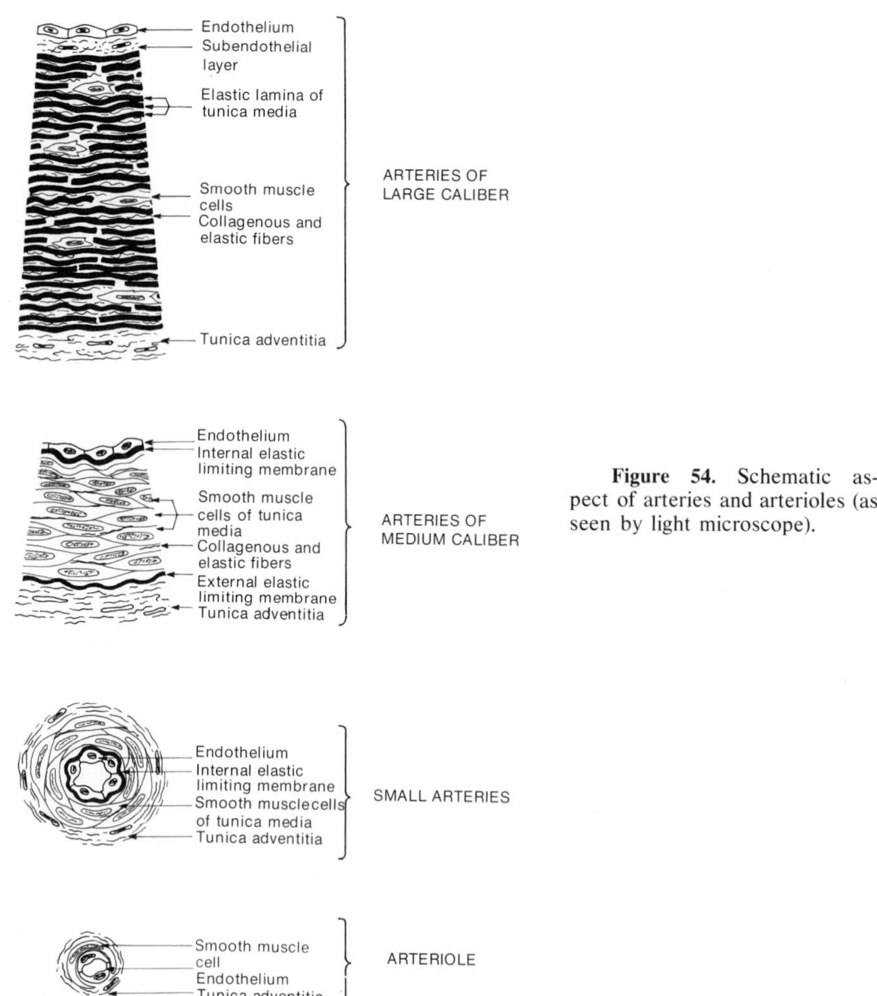

Figure 54. Schematic aspect of arteries and arterioles (as seen by light microscope).

B. ARTERIES

The arterial walls are composed of three concentric tunicae: (1) the tunica intima, facing the lumen, consisting of endothelium, basal lamina, and sometimes a subendothelial connective tissue layer; (2) the tunica media, made of smooth muscle cells and/or elastic tissue; and (3) an external tunica adventitia, made of connective tissue components.

Large arteries ("elastic arteries") are arterial trunks close to the heart (aorta, arteries of the neck, and pulmonary artery). Their elastic walls regulate the blood flow that is pumped rhythmically by cardiac systole.

Arteries of medium caliber ("muscular arteries") are found primarily in limbs and viscera. Contraction or relaxation of their walls increases or diminishes peripheral resistances, thus regulating blood flow of the various organs. Cerebral arteries possess a thin wall lacking a limiting external membrane, and a thin adventitia.

Some arteries (especially of the penis, uterus, bronchial tree, kidneys, and heart) have *blocking devices* which play an important role in regulation of blood flow. These devices are longitudinal fascicles of smooth muscle cells, located mainly in the tunica intima over a variable length (forming "rings," "tubes," "pads," or "little columns"), which temporarily occlude the vessel when contracting.

The walls of all arteries with a caliber of over 1 mm are supplied over at least two thirds of their exterior by vasa vasorum originating from the small arterioles that branch out in the area, or directly from the artery itself. The tunica intima and the inner area of the media appear to be nourished by imbibition from the blood circulating in the artery.

C. THE VEINS

Veins and venules have thinner walls and larger lumina than homologous arteries and arterioles. Their walls consist of an endothelium with its basal lamina resting on a more or less thick layer of connective tissue of collagenous fibers, fibroblasts, and varying numbers of elastic fibers. This connective tissue layer contains some smooth muscle cells, but their number, orientation, and location differ from one vein to another. On the whole, veins of the lower part of the body, which are under a high hydrostatic pressure, contain the most elastic fibers and smooth muscle cells; they also have numerous valves (endothelial folds containing collagenous and elastic fibers). Small venules have a structure very similar to that of the capillaries and, like them, are sites of exchanges between blood and tissues, especially in cases of inflammation. The walls of most veins have the capacity to contract actively, not only in order to maintain blood pressure in the highly distensible venous system but also to assist propulsion of blood in the vicinity of the heart.

The walls of veins are supplied by vessels penetrating from the tunica adventitia. Diffusion of nutritive substances from blood is negligible.

TABLE 20. Histology of Arterial Walls

Wall	Large Arteries (Elastic Arteries)	Medium Arteries (Muscular Arteries)	Small Arteries and Large Arterioles	Smallest Arterioles
TUNICA INTIMA				
Endothelium (simple squamous epithelium)	+	+	+	+
Basal lamina	+	+	+	+
Subendothelial connective layer	+	–	–	–
INNER ELASTIC LIMITING MEMBRANE	–	++	+	–
TUNICA MEDIA	Several layers of concentric fenestrated elastic fibers and some smooth muscle cells; some collagenous and elastic fibers	Numerous layers of smooth muscle cells arranged in a circle and some collagenous and elastic fibers	Some layers of smooth muscle cells arranged in a circle and some collagenous and elastic fibers	A single layer of smooth muscle cells arranged in a circle
EXTERNAL ELASTIC LIMITING MEMBRANE	–	+	–	–
TUNICA ADVENTITIA (Connective Tissue)	+	++	++	+ (Some fibroblasts and collagenous fibers)

D. THE HEART

The structure of the walls of the heart is analogous to that of the arteries, being composed of three layers—endocardium, myocardium, and epicardium—corresponding respectively to tunica intima, tunica media, and tunica adventitia of arteries.

I. Endocardium

Endocardium lines cardiac cavities and consists of endothelium resting on a connective tissue layer of variable thickness, which encloses adipose cells, small blood vessels, nerve fibers, and conduction system cells (bundle of His and its branches).

II. Myocardium

The myocardium consists of fascicles of cardiac muscle cells and conduction system cells. A meshwork of loose connective tissue, containing nerve fibers, lymphatics, and numerous blood capillaries, surrounds the cells or fascicles of muscle cells. The free ends of cardiac muscle cells are inserted into the "fibrous skeleton" of the heart (septum, fibrous trigone, and fibrous rings of the cardiac orifices).

III. Epicardium

The epicardium, covering the exterior of the heart, corresponds to the visceral pericardium, and is composed of a mesothelium resting on a connective tissue layer of varying thickness. Adipose cells, coronary vessels, and nerve fibers are embedded in the epicardium.

E. LYMPHATIC VESSELS

All organs, with the exception of the central nervous system, the inner ear, the bulbus oculi, and the bone marrow, contain lymphatic vessels.

I. Lymphatic Capillaries

Their structure is closely related to that of continous blood capillaries. They differ, however, inasmuch as they have a larger and more irregular lumen, they are blind-ending, and their basal laminae are of a discontinuous nature. The walls are surrounded by fascicles of reticular fibers bound to the outer side of the endothelial cells. These allow the opening of intercellular junctions by exerting traction, thus permitting the penetration of the interstitial fluid into the lymphatic capillaries.

II. Collecting Lymphatic Vessels

The structure of collecting vessels is similar to venules and veins of the same caliber. However, their walls are thinner than veins of the same caliber, and their valves are closer together.

The progression of lymph in these vessels is effected by rhythmic contractions of smooth muscle cells and by exterior forces (contraction of other muscle masses) which, applied to their walls, increase the intravascular pressure and produce a flow of lymph, with the valves serving to prevent reflux.

Lymphatic sinuses (or lymphatic sinusoid capillaries) are homologous with discontinuous blood capillaries. These exist only in lymph nodes.

13

Hematopoietic and Lymphoid Organs

A. LYMPH NODES

Lymph nodes are grouped in chains or aggregates along the course of lymphatic vessels, and drain adjacent areas via afferent lymphatics.

I. Connective Tissue Structure

The lymph node is partitioned by connective tissue trabeculae which penetrate from the capsule to the hilum. Afferent lymphatics penetrate the convex capsule at different points. Arteries enter the node at the hilum; veins and efferent lymphatic vessels exit from the hilum. Arteries and veins arborize into the trabeculae. At the periphery of the node, small venules play an important part in the recirculation of lymphocytes. In fact, blood lymphocytes can reach nodal tissue by passing between or through the endothelial cells of the venules.

II. Reticular Framework (stroma)

A delicate network of reticular fibrous tissue within the node differentiates to form the discontinuous wall of lymphatic sinuses. They separate the subcapsular sinus from intermediary sinuses, which form a complex

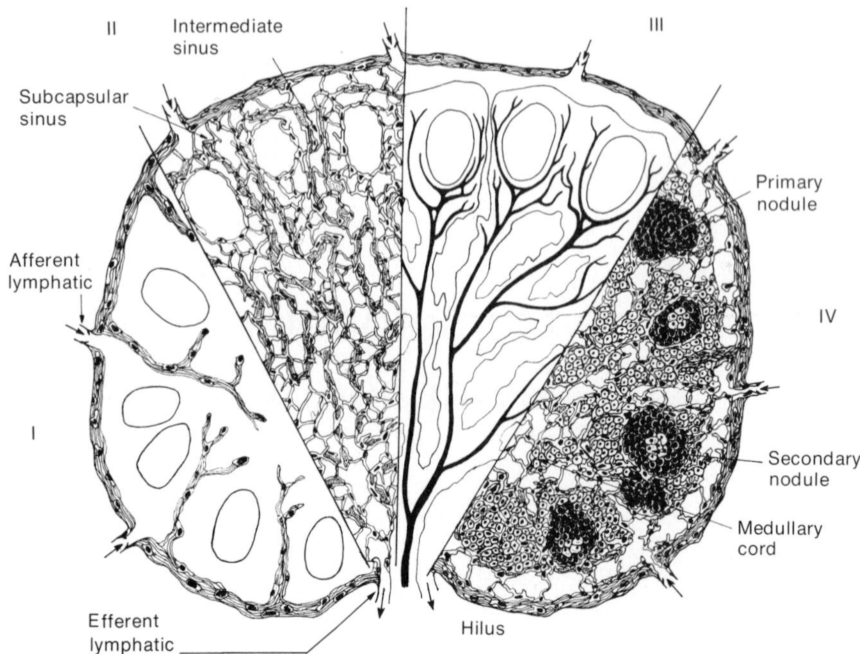

Figure 55. Diagram of a lymph node. *I,* Connective tissue stroma (framework). *II,* Reticular framework (delineates the lymphatic sinuses, partitions the node, and forms a network through the whole node). *III,* The venous distribution in the node, showing that postcapillary veins are located mainly in the cortex. *IV,* The free cells are grouped in nodules in the cortex and form cords in the medulla. (After L. Weiss, 1972.)

network in the central part of the node, and unite at the hilum to form efferent lymphatics.

This arrangement provides a remarkable filtration apparatus for lymph, especially for inanimate particles and bacteria, and a defensive mechanism against local and regional aggressions (mostly infectious). Its great efficiency is due to the fact that none of the elements of lymph returns to the venous circulation without having traversed at least one lymph node.

III. Free Cells

Cellular Equilibrium in the Nodes. Lymphoid cells, free macrophages, and some granulocytes are found in the meshes of reticular tissue. The relative proportions of these cell types depend on the functional condition of the lymph node (antigen stimulation).

Most lymphocytes form part of the circulating lymphocyte pool and, even though supplying lymphocytes to the lymph and blood is a function of the lymph node, the lymphopoietic capacity of the node is minimal under normal conditions. Macrophages form a relatively stable population, and none are found in efferent lymph. The population of plasma cells is also static, but precursors are found in the efferent lymph, and those can stimulate plasmocytopoiesis in other nodes.

Cellular Organization. Under the capsule free cells occur in great density, often forming primary or secondary lymphoid nodules. At the center of the node, cells form medullary cords, rich in plasma cells and macrophages. Between these two zones (cortex and medullary cord) an undelimited strip rich in small lymphocytes can be found. This zone, analogous to postcapillary venules, makes up the thymus-dependent zone of the node.

B. THE SPLEEN

The spleen is a lymphoid organ serving as a complex filter interposed in the course of the bloodstream.

I. Basic Structure (similar to lymph nodes)

Connective Tissue. Connective tissue makes up the capsule and the trabeculae delineating the lobules, which unite at the hilum, where veins and lymphatics also meet.

Reticular Fibers. These form a close mesh throughout the organ, and a dense anastomotic network of sinusoidial capillaries. The spleen has a filtration-purification function which, to its location, is effective in the defense against blood-borne noxious agents. As in the lymph node, filtration is both mechanical and biological (macrophage system). One of its classic tasks is the destruction of abnormal red blood corpuscles.

In the meshes of the reticular network, the following free cells are found: lymphoid cells, macrophages, and formed elements of the blood.

Free Cells. *Lymphoid cells* and *free macrophages* give evidence of the immunological capacity of the spleen and of the existence of lymphopoiesis and a plasmocytopoiesis. As in the lymph node, this cell population is not static, and the spleen lies in the path of cellular migrations which supply it with T lymphocytes (thymus-dependent areas) and B lymphocytes (bone marrow-dependent areas).

Formed elements of the blood include erythrocytes, granulocytes, and platelets. The spleen is a blood reservoir that maintains a regular flow to the portal veins supplying the liver. In the normal developing fetus (fifth to seventh month) and under certain pathological conditions, the spleen develops a myelopoietic capacity.

II. Particular Aspects Demonstrating the Structural Individuality of the Spleen

The Nature of its Vascularization. Upon leaving the trabeculae, arteries (the central arteries) enter the splenic tissue and branch out into numerous short collaterals to terminate in a group of penicillar arteries. These open into (1) the stroma of the reticular network and/or (2) the sinusoids, which anastomose to form the veins of the connective tissue trabeculae.

Opposed to this blood flow is a lymph flow, commencing in the venous sinuses and directed to efferent lymphatics which accompany the central arteries. This flow is important in the recirculation of small lymphocytes.

Free Cells. The free cells are organized around the vascular tree. Various arrangements permit several types of circulation, allowing certain cell elements to follow preferentially a given route.

White pulp is typically lymphoid tissue, cylindrical in form with a central artery as its longitudinal axis, with practically no formed blood elements. Lymphoid cells and macrophages form a periarterial lymphatic sheath with primary and/or secondary lymphoid nodules at certain points (Malpighian corpuscles).

Red pulp is formed by sinusoidal vessels with free cells surrounding them (cords of Billroth). Red pulp fills the spaces between the sinuses with components of circulating blood.

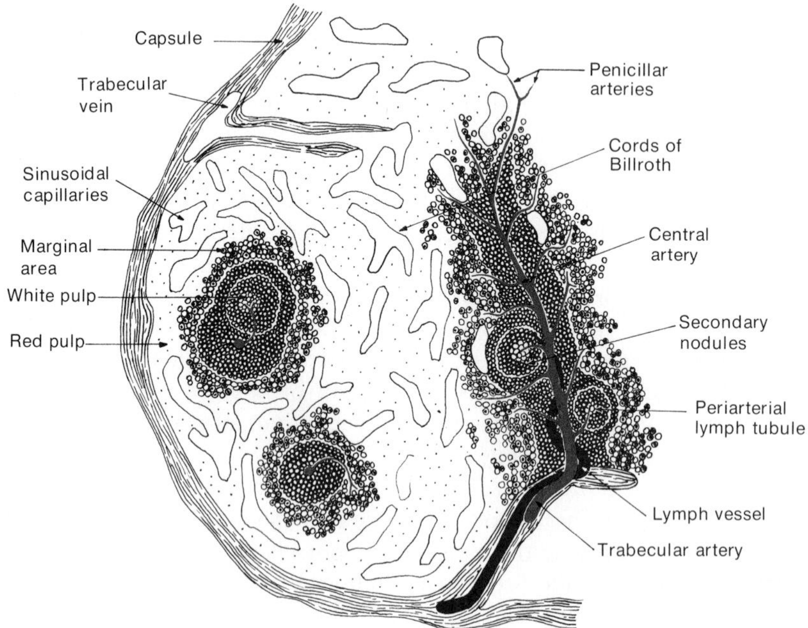

Figure 56. Diagram of the structure of the spleen (the cellular elements of red pulp are not shown).

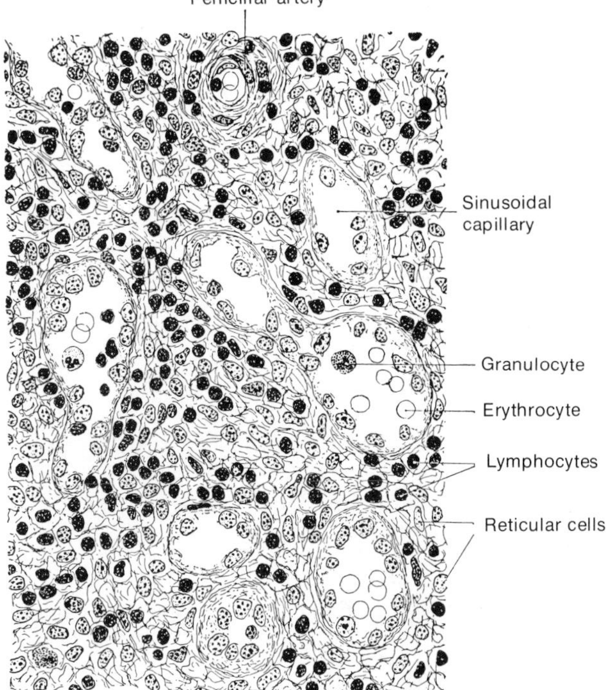

Figure 57. Red pulp of the spleen as seen with the light microscope (×500). (After O. Bucher, 1973.)

A marginal zone lies somewhere between red and white pulp, where nearly all collateral branches of the central artery terminate. It receives a large part of the blood perfusing the spleen and is the major site of cell differentiation and antigen concentration.

C. LYMPHOID FORMATIONS OF THE DIGESTIVE TRACT

Isolated lymphoid formations are located within diffuse lymphoid tissue which infiltrates the mucous membranes of the digestive tract. Their structure (lymphoid tissue plus reticular tissue) bestows on them a filtration-purification function against foreign elements in the interstitial fluid of the digestive mucosa, which is especially exposed to external contamination.

I. Tonsils

The palatine, lingual, pharyngeal, tubal, and laryngeal tonsils are masses of lymphoid tissue enclosed within the lamina propria of the mucous membrane of the area. The surface epithelium invaginates into this mass, forming the crypts which make up the tonsils.

II. Peyer's Patches

These are aggregations of primary and secondary lymphoid follicles located in the lamina propria of the terminal ileum.

III. Appendix

The lamina propria of the appendix is thickened by abundant lymphoid tissue over its entire circumference.

D. THYMUS

I. The Thymic Lobules

The thymus is a lymphoepithelial organ where certain lymphocytes proliferate and differentiate. The trabeculae originating from its connective

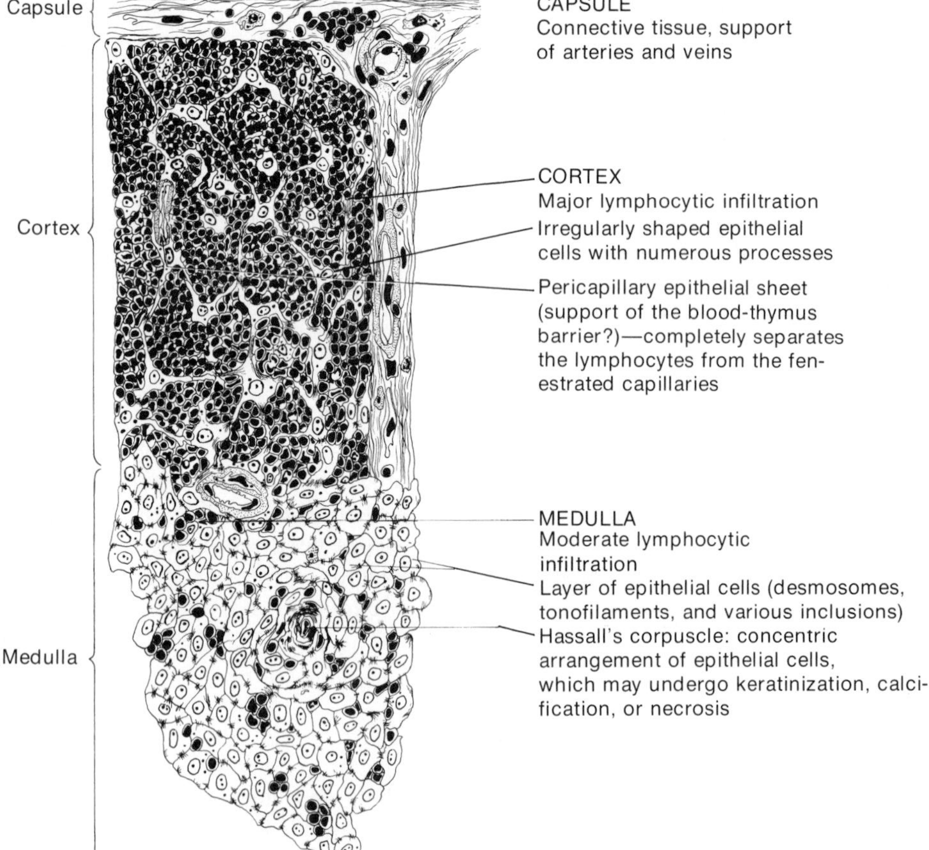

Figure 58. Portion of a thymic lobule. (After L. Weiss, 1972.)

tissue capsule divide into lobules, but separation is incomplete and the entire central area (medulla) forms an irregular but continuous column deep inside the organ.

The thymus, which is almost completely developed before birth, experiences a progressive involution during puberty, depleting it of lymphocytes and replacing the epithelial cells by adipose cells.

II. Thymic Lymphocytes or Thymocytes

The rate of production of thymic lymphocytes is very high. Ninety-five per cent of these lymphocytes have a short life span, developing and dying within the organ; the remaining 5 per cent have a long life span (T lymphocytes), and migrate from the thymus to colonize lymphoid organs. Lymphocyte production in these thymus-dependent areas could also be regulated by humoral factors secreted by epithelial cells. These "hormones" within the thymus have an influence on cell differentiation of lymphocytes, which become immunocompetent T cells.

Development and maintenance of the immune system depend on thymic lymphocytes. Experimental thymectomies have demonstrated their role in delayed hypersensitivity. The thymus in great measure controls the immune system, and therefore differs from other lymphoid organs. Among the distinguishing features are: Its development does not depend on any antigen stimulus, but it receives from bone marrow the permanent cells (undifferentiated lymphocytes) required to maintain lymphocyte production; it has no reticular network, no filtration function, and no macrophagic activity; and it contains neither lymphoid nodules nor plasma cells, and therefore no immunological reaction takes place there.

E. BONE MARROW

Bone marrow constitutes the central portion of bones. During development and throughout life it plays a major role in formation, growth, and modeling of bones. In the normal adult, it is the only myeloid organ and is the source of all lymphoid cells and free macrophages.

I. Vascular Components

Marrow is organized around blood vessels. Sinusoidal capillaries are important functional elements, forming a complex network with the reticular connective tissue throughout the marrow cavity. Bone marrow acts as a filtration-purification agent of the blood and serves as a destruction site of red corpuscles.

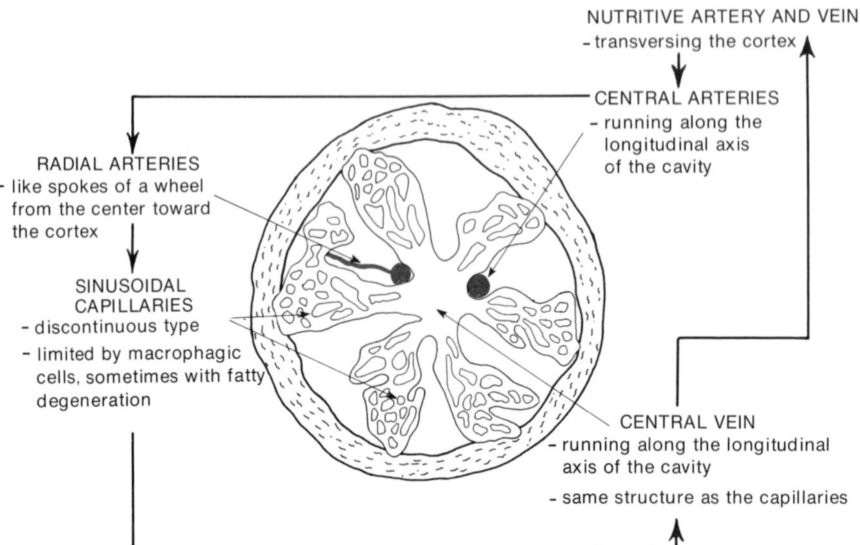

Figure 59. Vascular components of bone marrow.

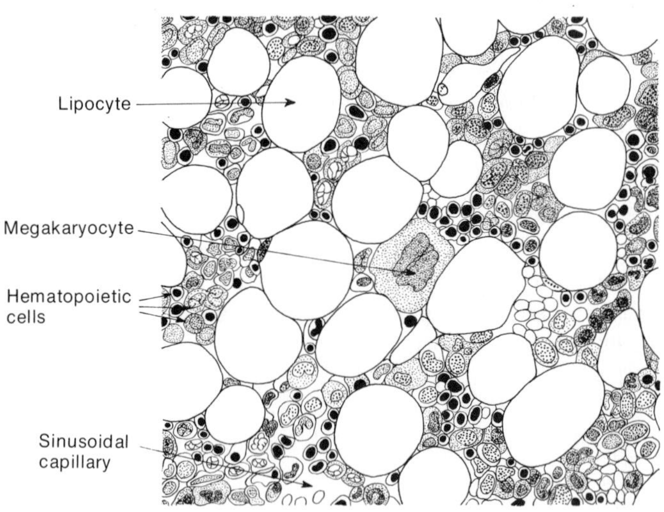

Figure 60. Bone marrow as seen with the light microscope (×550). (After W. Bargmann.)

TABLE 21. Cell Elements Observed in Bone Marrow

Cells	Location Within the Hematopoietic Tissue	Quantities
ERYTHROCYTES AND PRECURSORS	Often next to the walls of capillaries Erythroblastic islet: erythroblastic elements surround a macrophage	Three to four times less numerous than the elements of granulocytic lineage Erythrocyte reserve of about three times the total amount in the blood
GRANULOCYTES AND PRECURSORS	Often at a distance from the capillaries	Granulocyte reserve of more than 30 times the amount of circulating granulocytes
MEGAKARYOCYTES AND PRECURSORS	Near the walls of capillaries, where they discharge platelets into the lumen	
LYMPHOID ELEMENTS AND PRECURSORS	Scattered among other cells; possible formation of lymph nodes	Twenty per cent of the nucleated elements in the marrow
MONOCYTES AND MACROPHAGES	Disseminated and occurring in all capillaries	
STEM CELLS	Cannot be identified morphologically (probably of the lymphocytic type)	

TABLE 22. Schematic Representation of the Interrelations Between Vascular and Hematopoietic Components of the Bone Marrow

		STRUCTURE	
	LOCATION	*Sinusoidal Capillaries*	*Hematopoietic Components*
Red Marrow	Flat bones: ribs, vertebrae, sternum, cranial bones, ilium	Discontinuous wall permitting infiltrations and passage of cell elements	Developed; active hematopoiesis
Yellow Marrow	Long bones of the limbs and some of the flat bones	Adipose cells appearing in the adventitia and later in the endothelial layer	Very limited; it is an adipose tissue

II. Hematopoietic Components

Between the vascular components are found heterogeneous cell elements, indicating that marrow is an organ with an essential hematopoietic and immunological role.

Hematopoietic and vascular exchanges are selective; i.e., only mature elements of the different lineages leave the marrow under normal conditions.

III. Functional and Non-Functional Bone Marrow

There are great variations in the extent of the hematopoietic compartment, depending on the relative proportions of the sinusoidal capillaries, free cells, and lipocytes. A higher percentage of adipose tissue distinguishes yellow marrow from red marrow. Yellow marrow can become red and active again if required by altered conditions (physiological or pathological).

F. IMMUNE SYSTEM

Lymphoid tissue is responsible for immunological processes, and a remarkable functional organization can be observed in its different constituents.

Bone marrow is a complete hematopoietic and immunological organ. It is rich in stem cells and is the only organ for which a graft can correct the hematological and immunological effects of lethal radiation. Erythrocytes, polymorphonuclear cells, platelets, and precursors of macrophages and lymphoid elements develop and later colonize the marrow-dependent areas of the lymphoid organs (B lymphocytes and plasma cells).

The thymus is essential for the differentiation of T lymphocytes. These cells are immunologically competent and are responsible for reactions in cell immunity; they can also act as intermediaries in the production of antibodies.

Spleen, lymph nodes, and the lymphoid aggregations of the mucous membranes are made of a reticular framework containing cells from the marrow and the thymus that are capable of interacting with antigens, thus producing the complex reactions of cellular and humoral immunity. The spleen, which is interposed in the bloodstream, reacts mainly to antigenic stimuli from the blood (which are therefore systemic). Lymphoid formations, located in the pathways of the lymph and interstitial fluids, react to local aggressions.

Blood and lymph are circulating "immunological tissues" transporting antigens, active immunological cells, their precursors, and antibodies. They make possible exchanges between interdependent but widely dispersed lymphoid organs throughout the body. They support cellular migration and allow the diffusion of immune response, either amplifying a phenomenon that has started locally or permitting its acceleration when an antigen is reintroduced.

This organization makes it possible for a minimal quantity of antigens and cells, with immunological competencies specific to a particular antigen, to unite and engage all the immune system in an immune response.

14

Respiratory System

A. GENERAL STRUCTURE

I. Upper Respiratory Tract

Three types of mucosa are found in the cavities which conduct air from the exterior towards the trachea: nasal mucosa, olfactory mucosa, and buccopharyngeal mucosa.

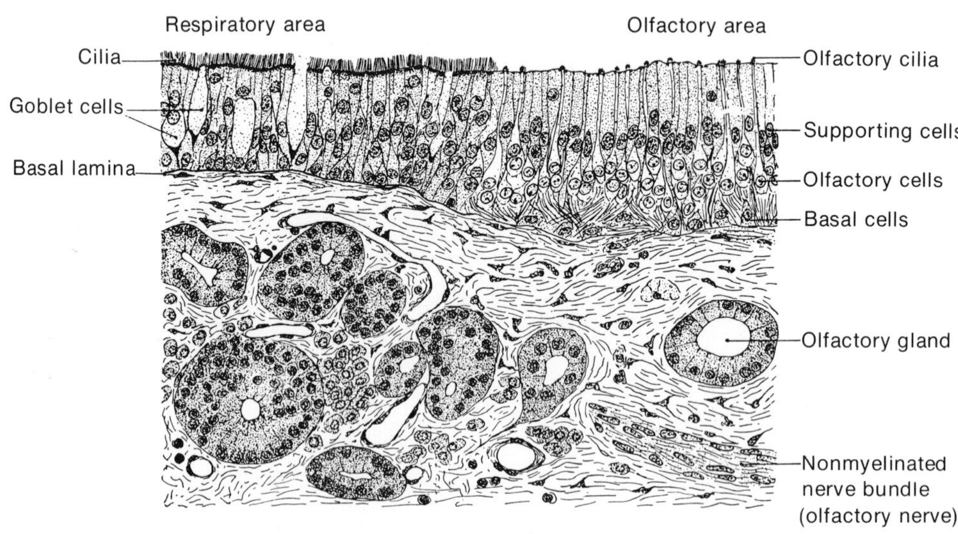

Figure 61. Nasal mucosa: junction of respiratory area and olfactory area (×250). (After O. Bucher, 1973.)

TABLE 23. Histology of the Upper Respiratory Tract

		Nasal Mucosa	Olfactory Mucosa	Buccopharyngeal Mucosa
ANATOMICAL LOCATION		Most of the nasal cavity; facial sinuses; nasopharynx; most of the larynx	Small area located at the upper inner part of the nasal cavities	Buccal cavity and tongue; oropharynx; anterior and superior part of the posterior side of the epiglottis; vocal cords
FUNCTION		Purification of inspired air	Olfaction	Protection of areas which come into contact with food
EPITHELIUM		Pseudostratified, ciliated columnar; mucous goblet cells	Pseudostratified columnar; olfactory neurosensory cells; supporting cells; basal replacement cells	Stratified squamous (nonkeratinized)
LAMINA PROPRIA	Glands	Nasal glands (ramified seromucosa)	Bowman's glands (tubuloacinous mucosa)	Small salivary glands
	Blood Vessels	+++ (large venous plexus)	++	+
	Nerves	Sensitive nerve endings	Sensitive nerve endings; fibers of the olfactory nerve (unmyelinated)	Sensitive nerve endings
	Lymphoid Tissue	++	±	++

II. The Lungs

Lungs are composed of (1) air conducting tubes, conveying air; (2) blood vessels, transporting blood; and (3) a connective interstitial tissue uniting both.

Air Conducting Tubes. During embryonic development, the respiratory diverticulum (from the foregut) gives rise, through successive branching, to 23 generations of branches of progressively decreasing length and thickness, to form the tracheobronchial tree (Table 24).

Blood Vessels (see Fig. 62).

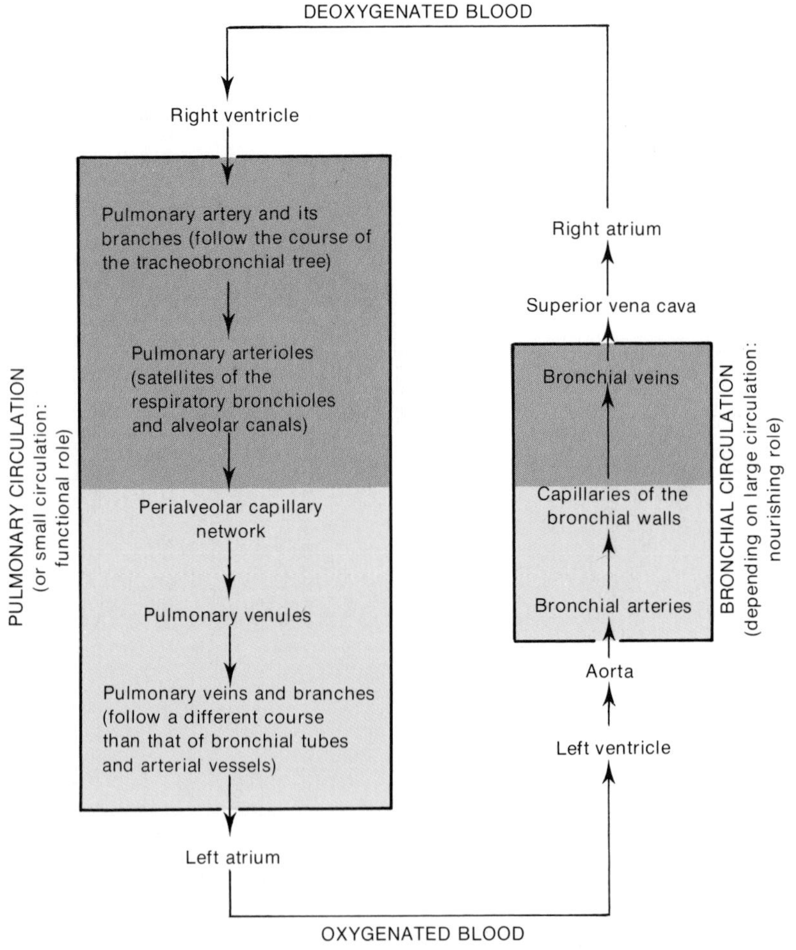

Figure 62. Blood vessels of the lungs.

Interstitial Tissue. This connective tissue joins the air and blood conducting systems to form the lungs. It makes up the connective tissue of large and medium bronchial ducts, arteries, and veins, the connective tissue sheaths of the pulmonary bronchioles and arterioles, and the connective tissue of the interalveolar septa. It also forms the interlobular walls, which continue at the periphery of the lungs as the subpleural connective tissue layer. The collagenous component confers solidity on the lungs. The elastic components (elastic fibers of the bronchial and arterial walls) contribute to the passive return of the lungs to the expiratory state after active dilatation initiated by the inspiratory muscles. Lastly, this interstitium supports the lymphatic system and nerves.

B. ALVEOLOCAPILLARY BARRIER

I. Alveolar Covering

This is a simple epithelium resting on a basal lamina and comprising two types of cells.

Small Alveolar Cells (Pneumonocytes Type I). These are the most numerous. Their flattened cytoplasm forms a thin wall extending from the

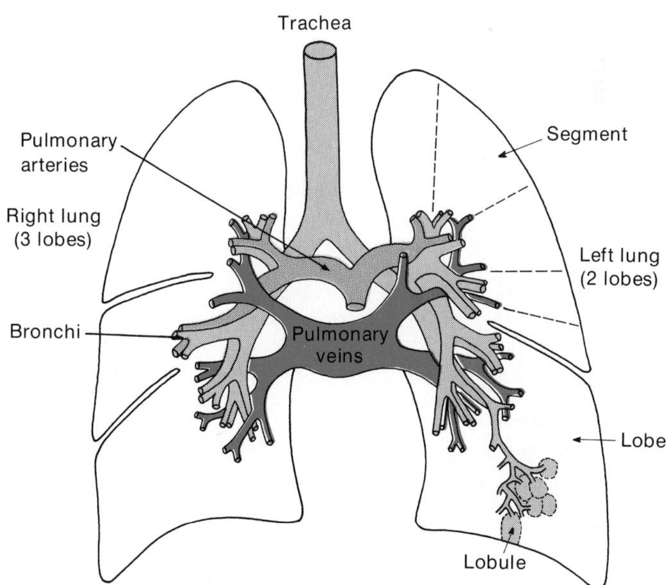

Figure 63. Diagram of the organization of air conducting tubes and blood vessels of the lungs. (Modified and redrawn after E. R. Weibel, 1963.)

TABLE 24. Histology of the Air Conducting Tubes of the Lungs

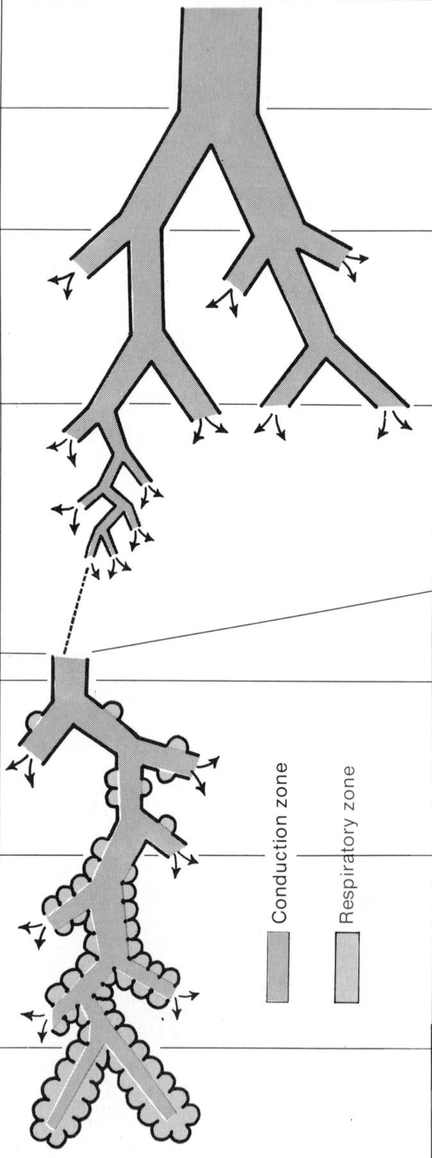

AIR CONDUCTING TUBES			
	Generation	*Dichotomy*	
Conduction Zone	0		Trachea (serving two lungs)
	1		Stem bronchi (each serving one lung)
	2 3		Interpulmonary bronchi (each serving one lobe, then a segment and a subsegment)
	4 5 6 7 8 ↓		Bronchioles (serving a pulmonary lobule)
	16		Terminal bronchi
Transition Zone And Respiratory Zone	17 18 19		Respiratory bronchioles (serving one pulmonary acinus)
	20 21 22		Alveolar canals
	23		Alveolar sacs

TABLE 24. *(Continued)*

Constitution of Their Walls					
Mucosa		*Smooth Muscle Cells*	*Glands*	*Hyaline Cartilage*	*Alveoli*
Epithelium	*Lamina Propria*				
Pseudostratified columnar; ciliated cells and goblet cells	Connective tissue rich in elastic fibers and lymphoid tissue	Tracheal muscle (uniting the posterior extremity of the cartilaginous arcs)	Tracheal glands (mucous and serous)	Cartilaginous arcs open at the back	
		Circular muscle	Bronchial glands (mucous and serous)	Irregular cartilaginous islets	
Simple columnar; ciliated goblet cells	Progressive diminution	Progressive diminution			
Simple cuboidal; lacking goblet cells; few ciliated cells					Some alveoli
Some nonciliated cuboidal cells	Some connective cells, and some collagenous and elastic fibers	Some smooth circular muscle			Numerous alveoli, leaving only alveolary outpouchings in the walls
"Alveolar Outpouchings"					
					Walls made of alveoli only

thicker area where the nucleus bulges, and contains numerous micropinocytotic vesicles.

Great Alveolar Cells (Pneumonocytes Type II). These are cuboidal in shape, have an apical pole with microvilli, and contain lamellar osmiophilic bodies which are secretion granules of surfactant. Surfactant is a lipoprotein which spreads on the surface of the alveoli, forming a thin film of surface active material that lowers surface tension and is essential for maintaining the stability of the alveoli.

II. Blood Capillaries

These are continuous, nonfenestrated capillaries surrounded by a continuous basal lamina. They form an intricate network in the interalveolar walls.

III. Interstitium of the Interalveolar Walls

These are thin connective spaces containing some fibroblasts and macrophages, as well as collagenous and elastic fibers, but *no* smooth muscle cells, lymphatic capillaries, or nerves. At certain points, there are "alveolar pores" which permit communication between adjacent alveoli.

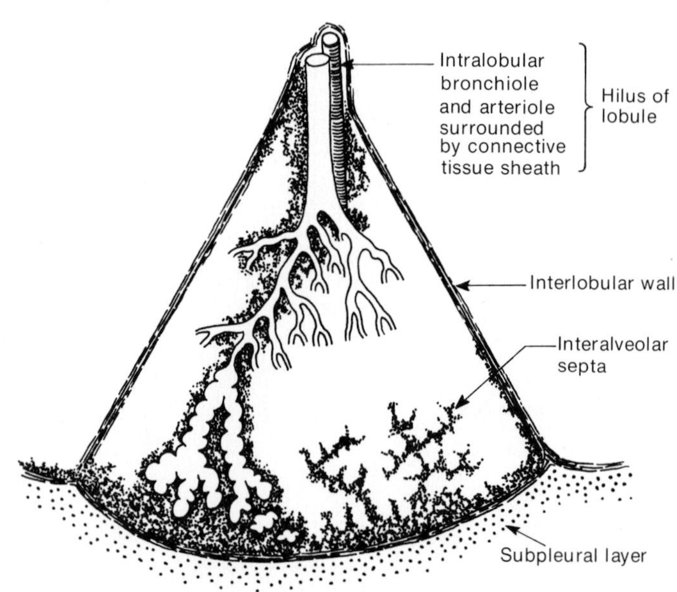

Figure 64. Pulmonary interstitium.

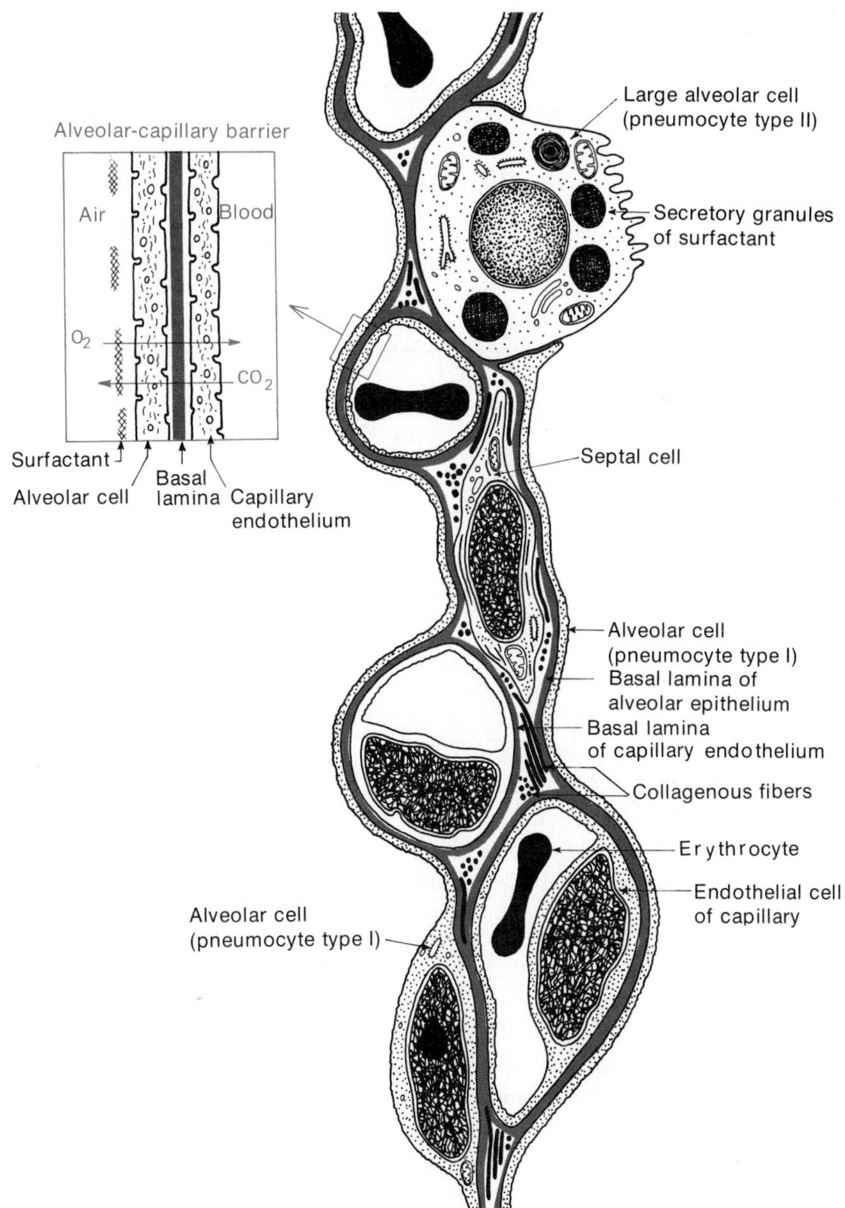

Figure 65. Alveolocapillary barrier.

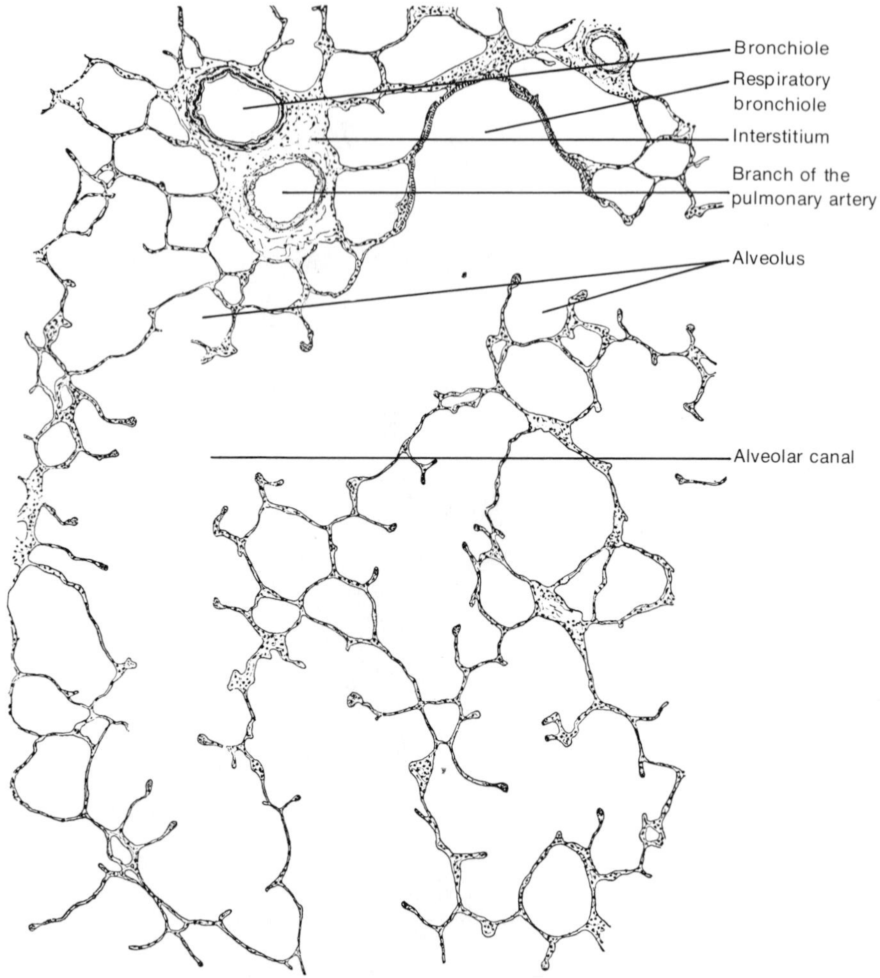

Figure 66. Lung (human), × 50. (After O. Bucher, 1973.)

IV. Gas Exchange

Gas exchange (O_2 and CO_2) between air and blood occurs by diffusion through the alveolocapillary barrier formed by the back-to-back abutment of small alveolar cells and capillary endothelial cells covered by a continuous basal lamina. At this level, the interstitium is extremely diminished.

C. PURIFICATION OF INSPIRED AIR

Beginning at the level of the nasal mucosa, inspired air is purified primarily by the mucociliary tracheobronchial apparatus and the alveolar macrophages.

I. Mucociliary Tracheobronchial Apparatus

The cilia of the tracheobronchial epithelium are blanketed by mucus produced by goblet cells and mucous glands. "Pushed toward the buccopharyngeal area by the coordinated movement of cilia, this mucous covering carries with it those particles that fall on it. With this mucous support, they reach the pharynx to be swallowed or expectorated" (Policard and Galy, 1970).

II. Alveolar Macrophages

Alveolar phagocytes (dust cells) differentiate from lymphocytes and/or monocytes after having passed through the alveolar wall. These are free cells in the alveolar cavity with phagocytic action on inorganic particles (dust) and organic particles (bacteria, spores, pollen, and so forth) which ciliary activity was not able to screen out. After phagocytosis is accomplished, macrophages can (1) reach the bronchioles to be evacuated by the ciliary apparatus, (2) degenerate in the alveoli, or (3) penetrate the interalveolar walls to reach lymph vessels and nodes occurring along their course.

15

Digestive System

A. BUCCAL CAVITY

The buccal cavity (as well as the oropharynx) is covered by a mucous epithelium of the nonkeratinized, stratified squamous type.

I. The Teeth

Each tooth consists of four types of tissue. Beginning with the innermost, these are: dental pulp, dentin, enamel, and cementum.

Dental Pulp. *Dental pulp is a loose connective tissue containing blood vessels and nerves.* It is confined within the pulp cavity (located within the tooth crown), which narrows into a dental canal opening at the roots. At the periphery, the pulp is bounded by a layer of cells (odontoblasts) originating in the mesenchyma.

Dentin. *Dentin surrounds the dental pulp.* Dentin is a ground substance produced by odontoblasts, which becomes calcified. Small tubules perpendicular to the surface traverse the dentin and contain cytoplasmic processes of the odontoblasts (Tomes' fibers).

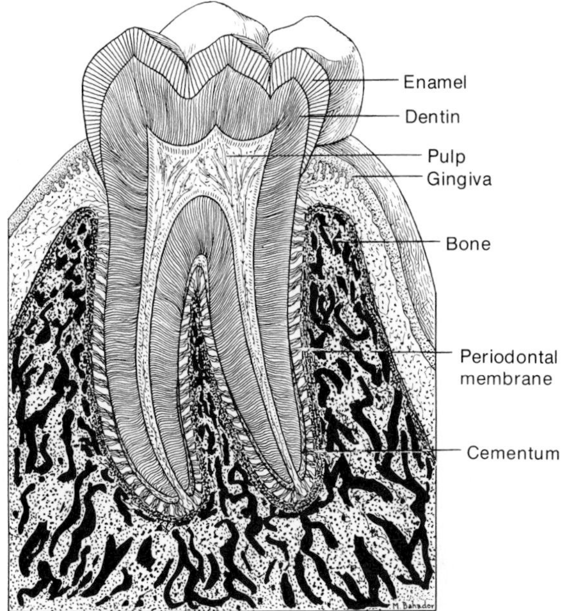

Figure 67. Diagram of a sagittal section of a molar in an adult. (After I. Schour in W. Bloom and D. W. Fawcett, 1975.)

Enamel and Cementum. *Enamel crowns the exposed exterior of the tooth, and cementum surrounds the roots.*

a. *Enamel,* the hardest substance in the body (97 per cent calcium salts) is secreted by ameloblasts during the intrauterine life. It is made of hexagonal prisms grouped in bundles with a grossly radial course, kept together by an interprismatic substance.

b. *Cementum,* made up of cells, collagenous fibers, and a calcified ground substance, is a variety of bone tissue.

II. Salivary Glands

These are exocrine, acinous, or tubulo-acinous glands having a mucous or serous secretion, or both.

Accessory Salivary Glands

Occurring almost everywhere in the mucosa of the buccal cavity and of the tongue, these glands have a short excretory canal with few or no branches, and a secretory portion made of mucous, serous, or seromucous acini or tubular acini, capped by myoepithelial cells.

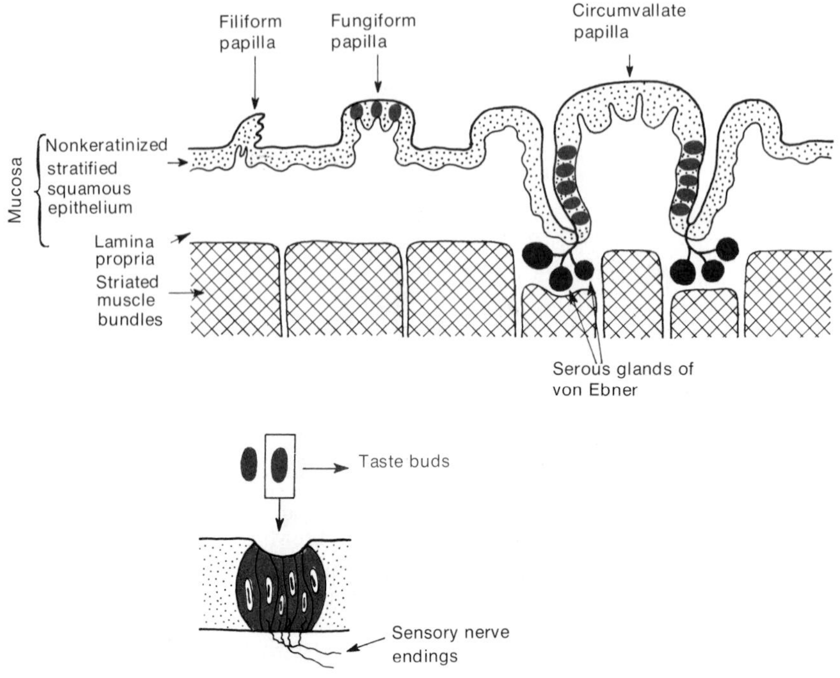

Figure 68. Lingual papillae.

Principal Salivary Glands

These glands have discrete anatomical characteristics. They contain lobules with long and highly branched excretory ducts–intralobular ducts draining into interlobular ducts and finally collecting ducts. The secretory portion is composed of acini or tubular acini (surrounded by myoepithelial cells). In the parotid gland, the acini are entirely serous; in the submandibular gland the acini may be mucous but are predominantly serous and mixed seromucous; in the sublingual gland the acini are occasionally serous but predominantly mucous and mixed seromucous.

Saliva

It is a product resulting from the secretion of all of these glands, and thus contains both mucus and enzymes (especially amylase).

III. The Tongue

The tongue consists of a central mass of striated muscle cells running in three planes and crossing at right angles. This striated muscular mass is covered by a mucosa having a structure identical to that of the rest of the buccal mucosa and contains numerous accessory salivary glands (anterior lingual glands, glands of von Ebner, glands of the root of the tongue).

Lingual Papillae

These are of four types.

a. *Filiform papillae,* the most numerous, are distributed over the anterior two thirds of the tongue. They are outgrowths of the lingual epithelium, with a core of connective tissue arising from the lamina propria.

b. *Fungiform papillae,* less numerous and occurring along the sides of the tongue, are larger outgrowths with a connective tissue core.

c. *Circumvallate papillae,* about 10 in number, are arranged along the V-shaped division between anterior two thirds and posterior one third of the tongue. They are larger than the fungiform papillae but have the circular furrow around the papilla. Glands of von Ebner open into the bottom of this furrow.

d. *Foliate papillae,* which occur on the lateral surface, but are less pronounced in humans than in other mammals (e.g., rabbit).

Taste Buds

The taste buds are located in the epithelium of the superior border of fungiform papillae and in the epithelium of the lateral faces of circumvallate and foliate papillae.

IV. Tonsils (see chapter 13)

B. DIGESTIVE TRACT

I. General Description

The walls of the digestive tract, from the esophageal opening to the anal orifice, consist of four concentric layers. Beginning with the outermost, these are (1) the tunica serosa (or adventitia), consisting of connective tissue; (2) the tunica muscularis, made up of smooth muscle cells; (3) the submucosa, made up of connective tissue; and (4) the mucosa, consisting of muscularis mucosae, lamina propria, and an epithelium facing the lumen.

At each anatomical level of the digestive tube, these four layers present particular morphological characteristics, which depend essentially on the (1) nature of the covering epithelium, (2) the nature and location of the various glandular formations of the mucosa and/or submucosa, and (3) the arrangement of the smooth muscles of the muscularis.

In addition to its main role of digestion, carried out by its epithelial lining (absorption of food), by its glands (protection and lubrication of the walls and degradation of food), and by its smooth muscles (peristalsis and mechanical mixing of the food), the digestive tube plays a role in defense (lymphoid formations) and secretes hormones (specific endocrine cells).

II. Epithelial Lining of the Lumen of the Digestive Tube

Three types of epithelia line the inside of the digestive tube:

Epithelium for Mechanical Protection

This lining occurs at the two extremities of the digestive tube (esophagus and anal canal) and consists of stratified squamous epithelium. It is nonkeratinized in the esophagus and over the upper third of the anal canal; it is keratinized over the lower two thirds of the anal canal and continues into the skin of the anal margin.

Epithelium for Chemical Protection

This type occurs only in the stomach and consists of a simple columnar epithelium with cells with short microvilli. The mucous secretion supplied by this secretory epithelium contributes to the lubrication of the gastric wall, and to protection against damage from harsh gastric juices.

Absorptive Epithelium

This lines the whole length of the intestine, from duodenum to rectum. It is a simple columnar epithelium with a striated border, and numerous goblet cells.

a. *The goblet cells* contribute to the lubrication of the intestinal lumen with their mucous secretion.

b. *The enterocytes (intestinal epithelium)* are characterized by a great absorptive capacity owing to the numerous microvilli at their apical poles. The microvilli are arranged parallel to each other, making up the striated border seen with the light microscope.

Absorption of Proteins and Carbohydrates. A great number of hydrolytic enzymes (peptidases, aminopeptidases, disaccharidases, alkaline phosphatases, and so forth) are found at the striated border of the enterocytes, either in the plasmalemma of the microvilli (which is the case for enzymes synthesized by the cell) or in the meshes of the glycocalyx around microvilli (enzymes in chyme and in pancreatic juices, which are then absorbed at the surface of the enterocyte). These diverse enzymes are responsible for the final stages in the hydrolysis of the proteins and carbohydrates in food, and thus deliver amino acids and glucose to the "transporters" of the plasmalemma, which convey them to the interior of

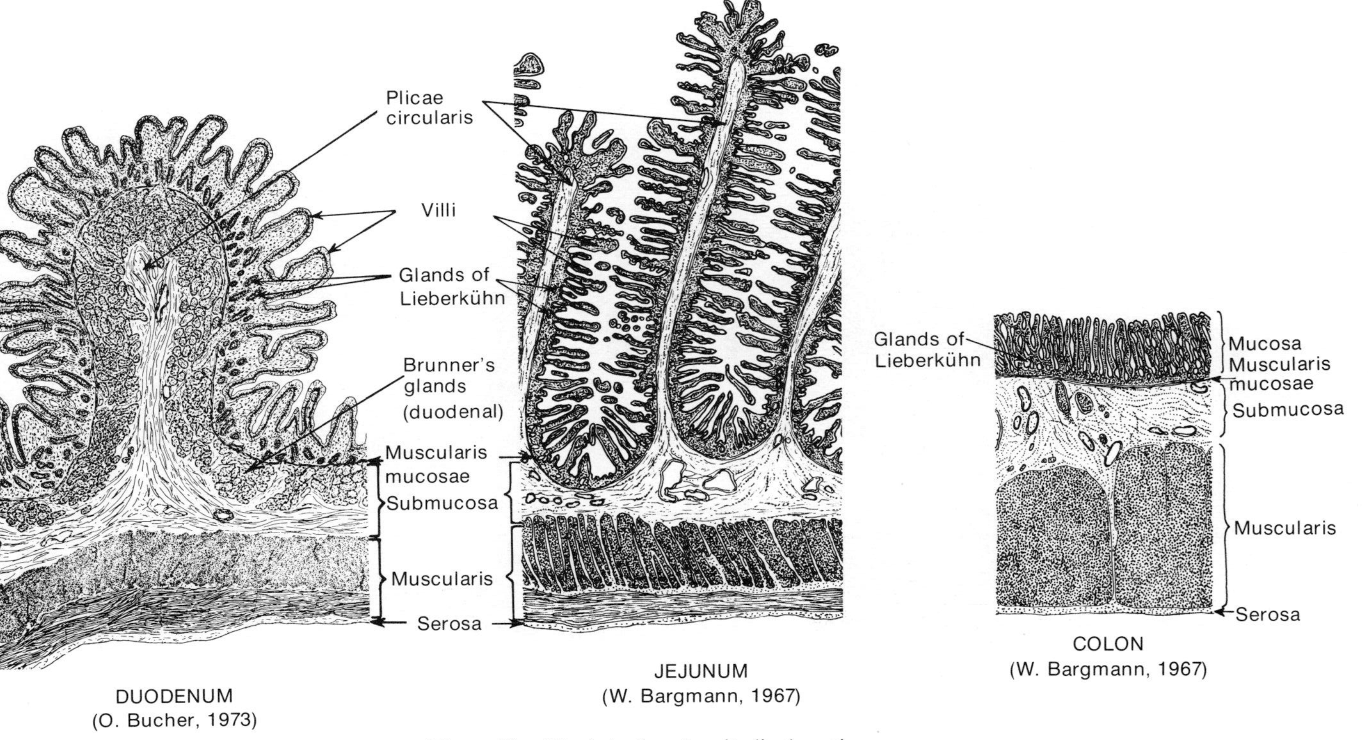

Figure 69. The intestine: longitudinal sections.

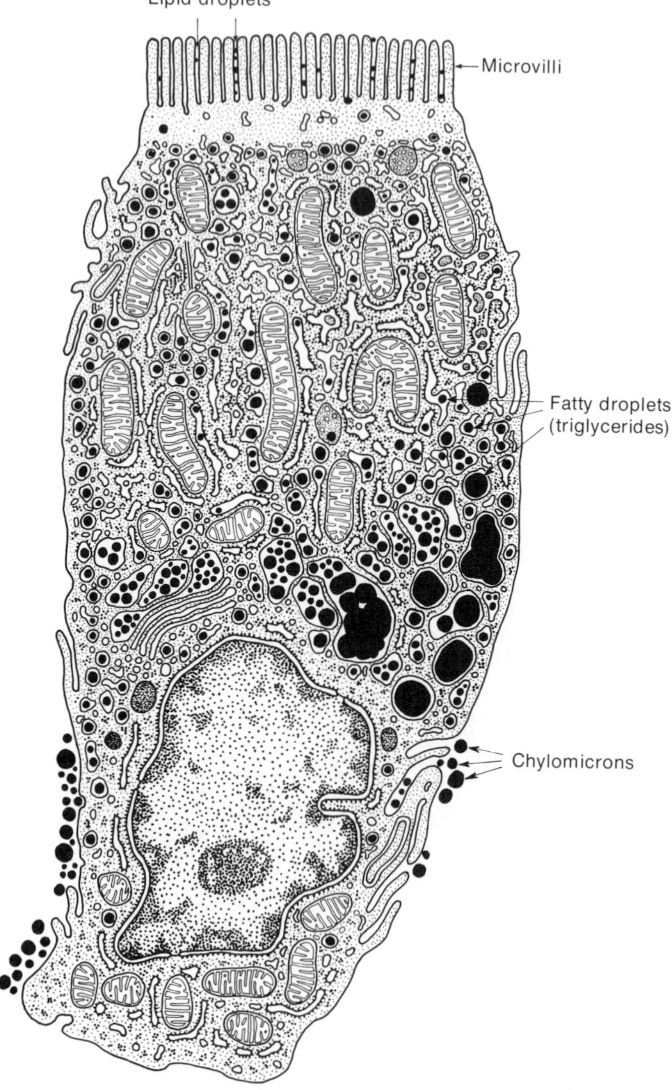

Figure 70. Absorption of fats in an enterocyte (as seen by electron microscopy). (After T. L. Lentz, 1971.)

the enterocytes. From there they are released into the underlying blood capillaries.

Absorption of Fats. Triglycerides (which make up more than 98 per cent of ingested fats) are hydrolyzed in the intestinal lumen by pancreatic lipase into free fatty acids and monoglycerides. These conjugate with bile salts to form a solution of lipid droplets. The droplets of free fatty acids and monoglycerides diffuse passively through the microvilli, and are incorporated into the endoplasmic reticulum, where they resynthesize triglycerides, which appear as fat droplets. These are released into intercellular spaces as chylomicrons by the smooth endoplasmic reticulum, and later reach the lymphatic capillaries.

In the small intestine (duodenum, jejunum, and ileum) enterocytes are more abundant than goblet cells. Their striated border of microvilli augments the already large absorptive surface consisting of:

1. *Intestinal loops* or coils.
2. *Plicae circulares* (permanent transverse folds of the mucosa and the muscularis mucosae).
3. *Intestinal villi* (finger-like projections of the mucosa, with a connective tissue core containing smooth muscle cells, an arteriole branching out into a capillary network drained by a venule, and a blind-ending lymphatic capillary).
4. *The microvilli of the enterocytes.*

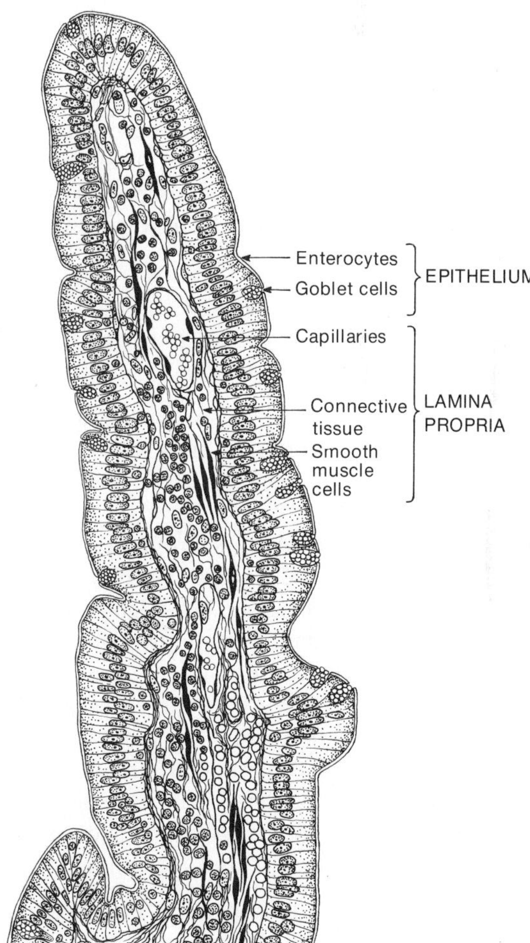

Figure 71. Intestinal villi (×400). (After W. Bargmann, 1967.)

The extraordinary increase in surface area made possible by this complex apparatus demonstrates the essential role that the small intestine plays in absorbing the degradation products of food.

In the colon and rectum, goblet cells outnumber enterocytes, and intestinal loops, plicae circulares, and villi are lacking.

III. Exocrine Glands of the Digestive Tube

Numerous exocrine glands located in the lamina propria of the mucosa or submucosa of the wall of the digestive tube release their secretory products into its lumen.

Mucous Glands

Some of these glands secrete only mucus to lubricate and protect the walls of the digestive tube.

a. *The esophageal glands* are compound acinous glands located in the submucosa of the esophagus.

b. *The cardiac glands* are tubulo-alveolar glands located in the lamina propria of the mucosa at the lower extremity of the esophagus and at the upper extremity of the stomach.

c. *Pyloric glands* are short convoluted tubular glands located in the lamina propria of the pyloric antral mucosa.

d. *Brunner's glands* are compound tubulo-alveolar glands located in the submucosa of the duodenum (duodenal glands).

Other Glands

Other glands secrete not only mucus but also enzymes and/or HC1, which participate in the hydrolysis of food proteins and carbohydrates.

a. Fundic Glands. These are elongated, straight tubular glands with a narrow lumen. They open into the bottom of the epithelial crypts of the fundus and body of the stomach. These glandular tubes are made up of three cell types:

1. *Mucous neck cells,* secreting mucus.
2. *Chief cells,* the most numerous, have all the morphological characteristics of protein secreting cells. The enzymatic content of their secretory granules consists mainly of pepsinogen (proteolytic enzyme) and (in infants) rennin (milk coagulating enzyme).
3. *Parietal cells* are very large and appear to be pushed to the periphery of the glandular tubes by the chief cells between which they are wedged. Their main characteristics are an abundance of large round mitochondria, numerous small pale vesicles, and an intracellular network of canaliculi, formed by invaginations bordered by microvilli. They secrete hydrochloric acid, as Cl^- and H^+ ions, into the intracellular canaliculi.

b. The Glands (Crypts) of Lieberkühn. These glands are tubular glands located in the lamina propria of the small intestine mucosa and

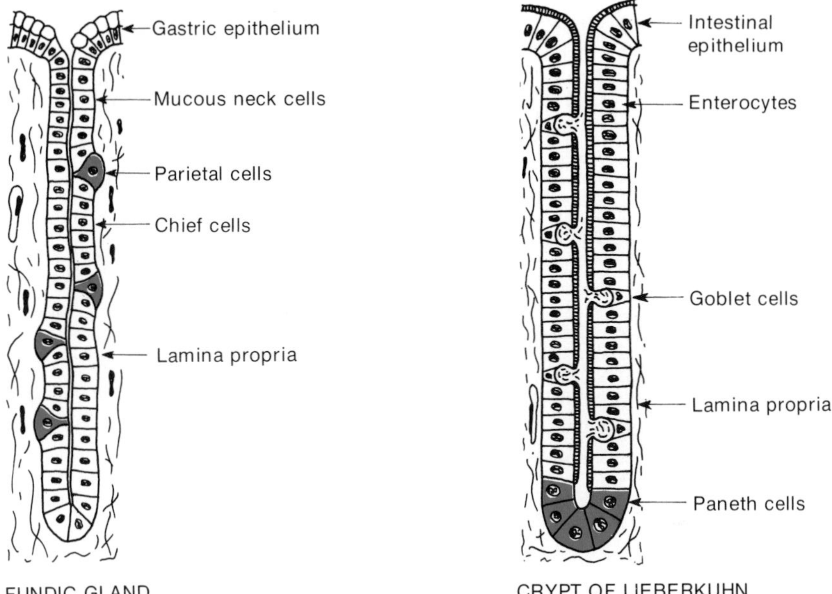

Figure 72. Fundic glands and crypts of Lieberkühn.

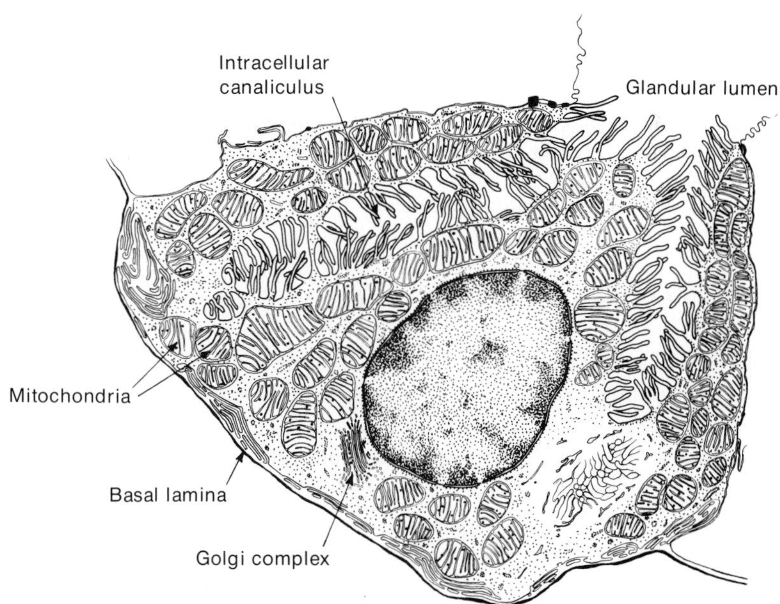

Figure 73. Diagram of a parietal cell (as seen with electron microscope). (After S. Ito and R. J. Winchester, 1963.)

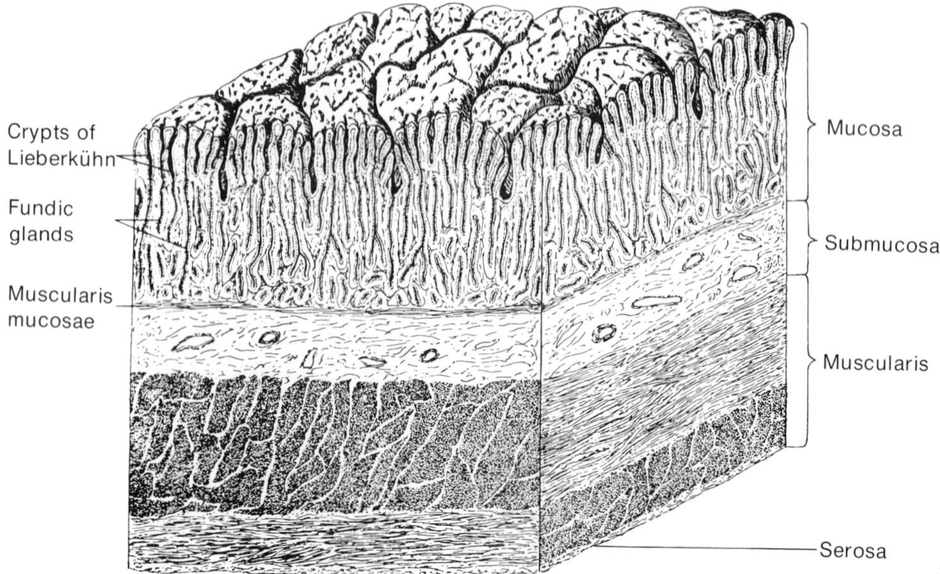

Figure 74. Gastric wall. (After O. Bucher, 1973.)

the colon and rectum. They are invaginations of the intestinal epithelium opening between the villi and consist mainly of enterocytes and large Paneth cells. The latter, located at the bottom of the glandular tubes, are characterized by all the organelles occurring in protein secreting cells, and by large secretory granules with an enzymatic content, of unknown nature.

In addition to glandular secretions, the intestinal lumen contains: (1) products of food degradation, (2) bile, (3) pancreatic juice, (4) plasma proteins leaking from the capillaries of the lamina propria, and (5) cellular waste material resulting from the rapid renewal of the intestinal epithelium.

IV. Endocrine Cells of the Digestive Tract

These cells, grouped under the general term of enterochromaffin cells (or argentaffin cells), are scattered in the epithelium of the digestive tract below the diaphragm, such as in the gastric gland epithelium and the intestinal crypts of Lieberkühn, but predominantly in the small intestine and appendix. The cells are wider at their basal poles and rest on the basal lamina; their slender apical poles may or may not reach the lumen of the tract or gland. Their cytoplasm is characterized by the presence of spherical granules that are visible only after using special stains (argentaffin reaction, chromaffin reaction, fluorescence). With the electron microscope, they appear as electron-dense membrane-bound granules surrounded by a light halo. All these cells release their secretory products into the blood. Some

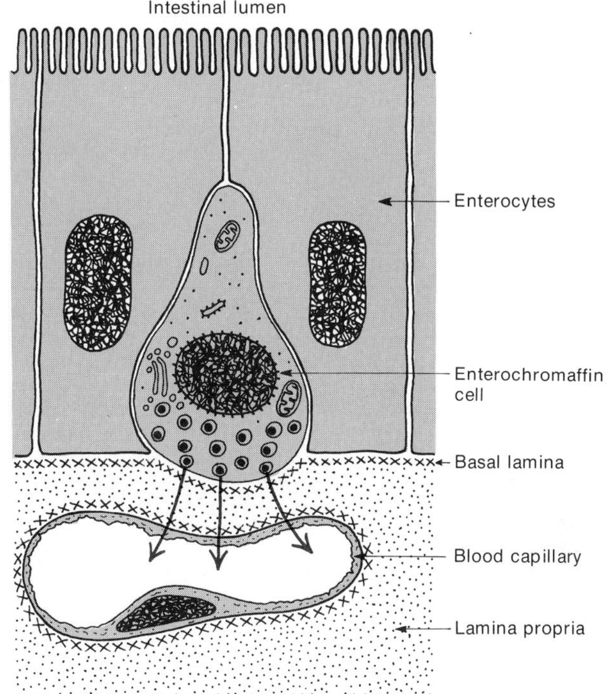

Figure 75. Schematic representation of an enterochromaffin cell as seen with the electron microscope.

secrete serotonin, and others, located in the pyloric glands, secrete gastrin. Still others secrete various hormones (secretin, cholecystokinin, pancreozymin, enterogastrone, enteroglucagon, and so forth), but the exact relationship between cells and hormones is not well defined.

V. Lymphoid Formations of the Digestive Tube

Diffuse lymphoid tissue occurs in the mucosa and sometimes in the submucosa throughout the digestive tract. In addition, three types of distinct lymphoid formations occur in tonsils, Peyer's patches of the ileum, and the appendix.

VI. Musculature of the Digestive Tube

The smooth musculature of the digestive tube, producing digestive motility, is usually composed of two layers: inner circular and outer longitudinal muscle layers. The thin muscularis mucosae is located between mucosa and submucosa. The nerve plexuses responsible for the extrinsic sympathetic and parasympathetic innervation are located in the submu-

TABLE 25. Histology of the Wall of the Digestive Tube

Digestive Tube		Mucosa	
		Epithelium	*Lamina Propria*
Esophagus		Nonkeratinized stratified squamous	Cardiac glands (mucous) at the upper and lower extremities
Stomach		Simple columnar with mucus-secreting cells	Gastric glands: Fundic glands in the body and fundus Pyloric glands in the antrum
Duodenum		Simple columnar with enterocytes having a striated border (+++) and goblet cells	Crypts of Lieberkühn; at base of the villi; lymphoid follicles (++); Peyer's patches (at the distal ileum)
Jejunum–Ileum			
Appendix		Simple columnar with goblet cells (+++) and enterocytes having a striated border	Crypts of Lieberkühn; lymphoid nodules (+++) especially in the appendix
Colon and Rectum			
Anal Canal	Ano-rectal Area	Nonkeratinized stratified squamous	Large venous plexus
	Ano-cutaneous Area	Keratinized stratified squamous	No distinguishing features
	Cutaneous Area		Pilosebaceous follicles and apocrine sweat glands

TABLE 25. ***(Continued)***

Muscularis Mucosae	Submucosa	Muscularis	Peripheral Connective Layer
Absent in the upper third; outer striated muscle in upper third	Esophageal glands (chiefly mucous, but also serous)	Two layers (inner circular and outer longitudinal); outer striated muscle in the upper third or half	Adventitia; serosa for subdiaphragmatic portion
Two layers with radial processes entering the mucosa	No distinguishing features	Three layers (inner oblique, middle circular, and outer longitudinal)	
Elevated by the plicae circularis	Brunner's glands (acinous mucous)	Two layers (inner circular and outer longitudinal)	Peritoneal serosa (except at the posterior contact points of the peritoneum—duodenum, colon, rectum)
	No distinguishing features		
Discontinuous	Lymphoid nodules (++)		
No distinguishing features	No distinguishing features	Two layers (inner circular and outer interrupted longitudinal) (colic bands)	
		Inner smooth muscle sphincter (thickening of the inner circular layer)	Adventitia
		Outer striated muscle sphincter	

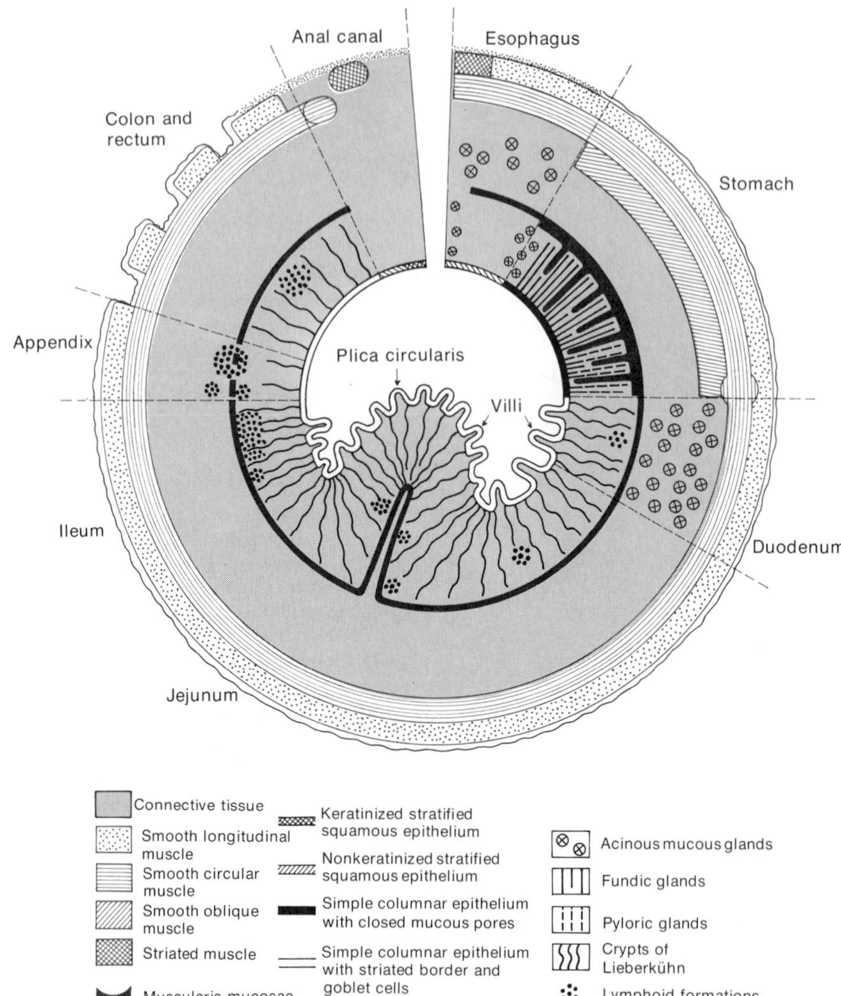

Figure 76. Diagram of the structure of the wall of the digestive tube.

cosa (Meissner's plexus), and between the two layers of the muscularis (Auerbach's plexus).

The muscularis and the muscularis mucosae present organizational differences depending on the level at which they occur. In the upper one third to one half of the esophagus, the outer longitudinal layer of the muscularis is made of striated muscle cells. In the stomach, the muscularis consists of three layers (inner oblique, middle circular, and outer longitudinal) and the muscularis mucosae branches out into folds perpendicular to the surface and wedged between the glands. In the colon, the outer longitudinal layer of the muscularis is discontinuous and forms three thickened narrow bands (teniae coli), which, owing to their relative shortness, are responsible for "colonic haustrae." In the anal canal, the inner circular layer thickens into a smooth muscular sphincter, and toward its distal end the muscularis disappears, to be replaced by a striated muscular sphincter.

C. LIVER AND BILIARY TRACTS

I. Parenchymal, Vascular, and Biliary Compartments

Whether considered anatomically (liver and bile ducts), histologically (hepatic tissue), or cytologically (hepatic cells), the liver can be viewed as comprising three compartments intimately linked by connective tissue.

II. Organization of These Three Sections

The Organ Level

The liver is surrounded by a connective tissue capsule which, at the porta hepatis, is continuous with the connective tissue arborization that accompanies the ramifications of the (1) extrahepatic bile tracts (which exit the liver here), and (2) the hepatic artery and the portal vein (both of which enter it). The superior hepatic vein exits the liver at its upper posterior side.

The Tissue Level

In a liver section viewed under low power, the hepatic parenchyma is seen to consist of rows of hepatic cells, or hepatocytes. These branching and anastomosing cell layers are surrounded by a network of sinusoidal blood capillaries bound by a thin mesh of reticular fibers. Within this parenchymal mass are hexagonal substructures called lobules, which are characterized by: (1) portal canals made up of a small branch of the hepatic artery, a branch of the portal vein, and a bile ductule, all invested in a common connective tissue sheath containing nerve and lymph vessels, and (2) the central veins, which drain into the hepatic veins. The arrangement of portal canals and central veins serves to distinguish several hypothetical structural or functional units: (1) the classic hepatic lobules, (2) portal lobules, and (3) hepatic acini.

The Cell Level

Each of the four lateral sides of an hepatocyte (considered schematically as a cuboidal cell) contacts adjacent hepatocytes of the same layer (delimiting the bile canaliculi), and the remaining two sides bound the sinusoidal blood capillaries which invest their reticular layer.

a. The Hepatocytes. Hepatocytes have a large nucleolated nucleus. Some cells are binucleate. The cytoplasm varies according to the functional condition of the cell and contains all the usual organelles, as well as masses of pigment (lipofuscin), lipid inclusions, and numerous glycogen granules. At the vascular poles of the hepatocytes, the plasmalemma has numerous microvilli where exchanges between hepatocytes and blood occur. These

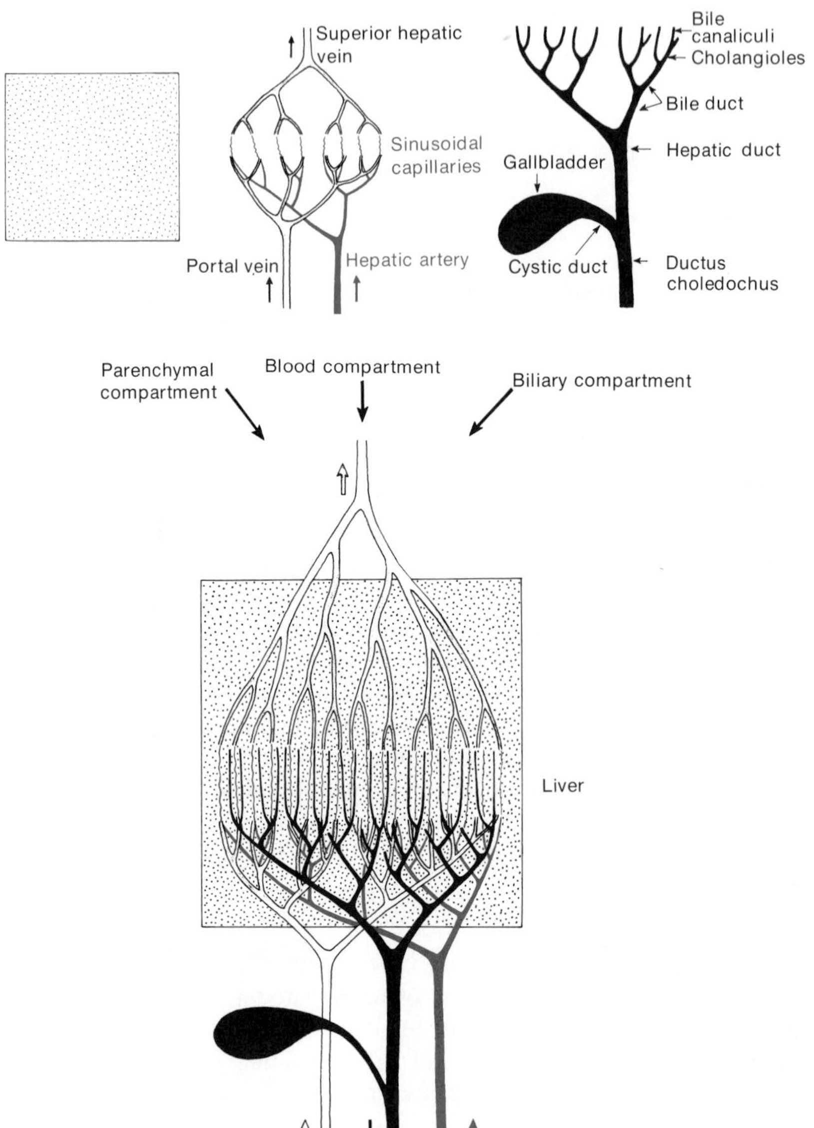

Figure 77. The three compartments of the hepatobiliary apparatus.

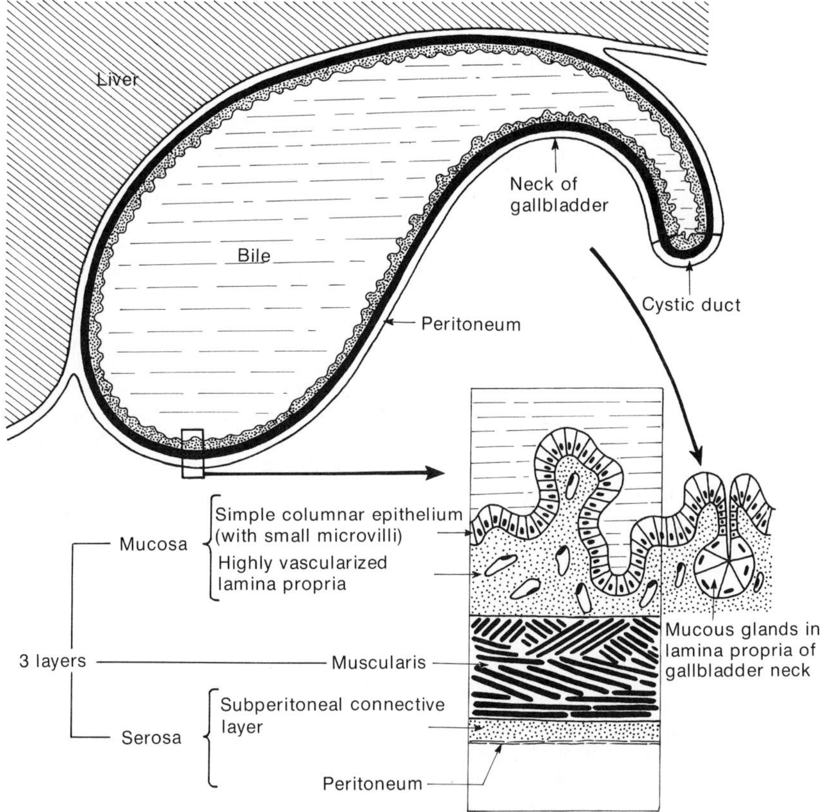

Figure 78. The gallbladder (1) *stores* bile secreted continuously by the liver; (2) *condenses* it (by reabsorbing water and electrolytes through its epithelium; (3) *releases* bile into the duodenum under the effect of certain stimuli (cholecystokinin, fatty foods); (4) *adds* mucus (through the mucous glands in the neck of the gallbladder.).

are very important exchanges, since the hepatic cell, with its extensive enzymatic capabilities and strategic situation in contact with blood from the digestive organs, participates in most of the intermediary metabolisms, among which are:

Carbohydrate metabolism (especially storage of blood glucose as glycogen and release of glucose into the blood by glycogenolysis). Most enzymes involved in carbohydrate metabolism occur free in the hepatocyte cytoplasm. Glycogen granules are usually localized within the zones of cells that are rich in smooth endoplasmic reticulum, but the significance of this close topographic relationship is not known.

Lipid metabolism. Synthesis of lipids associated with carbohydrates or proteins; synthesis of cholesterol; transformation of lipids into lipoproteins (chylomicrons). Smooth endoplasmic reticulum plays a fundamental role in lipid synthesis.

TABLE 26. The Hepatobiliary Apparatus

	Distribution Within Parenchyma			
Vascular Compartment	Afferent Vessels			Portal vein and its branches (ending as venules) = portal circulation (functional) Hepatic artery and its dividing branches (ending as arterioles) = systemic circulation (nutritive)
	Sinusoidal Capillaries			Receiving afferent vessels and draining into efferent vessels
	Efferent Vessels			Central veins → superior veins → inferior vena cava
Biliary Compartment	Intrahepatic Bile Ducts		Bile Canaliculi	Hexagonal network inside the layers of hepatocytes, between the hepatocytes, bounding them directly
			Cholangioles	Wall made up of simple cuboidal epithelium
			Biliary Canals	Wall made up of simple cuboidal epithelium (located in the portal spaces)
	Extrahepatic Bile Ducts	Chief Bile Ducts	Hepatic Duct	Wall made up of: A mucosa { Simple columnar epithelium; Lamina propria containing mucous glands } A smooth muscularis A serosa (peritoneum)
			Ductus Choledochus	
			Cystic Duct	
			Gallbladder	(See Fig. 78)

Protein metabolism (especially synthesis of plasma proteins, albumin, globulins, fibrinogen, prothrombin, and so forth). Ribosomes and granular endoplasmic reticulum form the morphological basis for protein synthesis.

Degradation of numerous liposoluble drugs (barbituric acids, for example) and of steroid hormones. The enzymes responsible for this phenomenon are located in the smooth endoplasmic reticulum.

At the biliary poles of hepatocytes, the plasmalemmas of adjacent hepatocytes indent to form bile canaliculi. Here the hepatic cells excrete salts and biliary pigments (bilirubin) synthesized by them.

b. Sinusoidal Blood Capillaries. Hepatic capillaries are large and irregular; their discontinuous walls are made up of a single layer of endothelial cells with more or less large interstices between them. There is no basal lamina, but some reticular fibers occur in a small space ("space of Disse") which separates sinusoids from surrounding hepatic cells (these are the fibers stainable with silver that form a feltwork corresponding to the

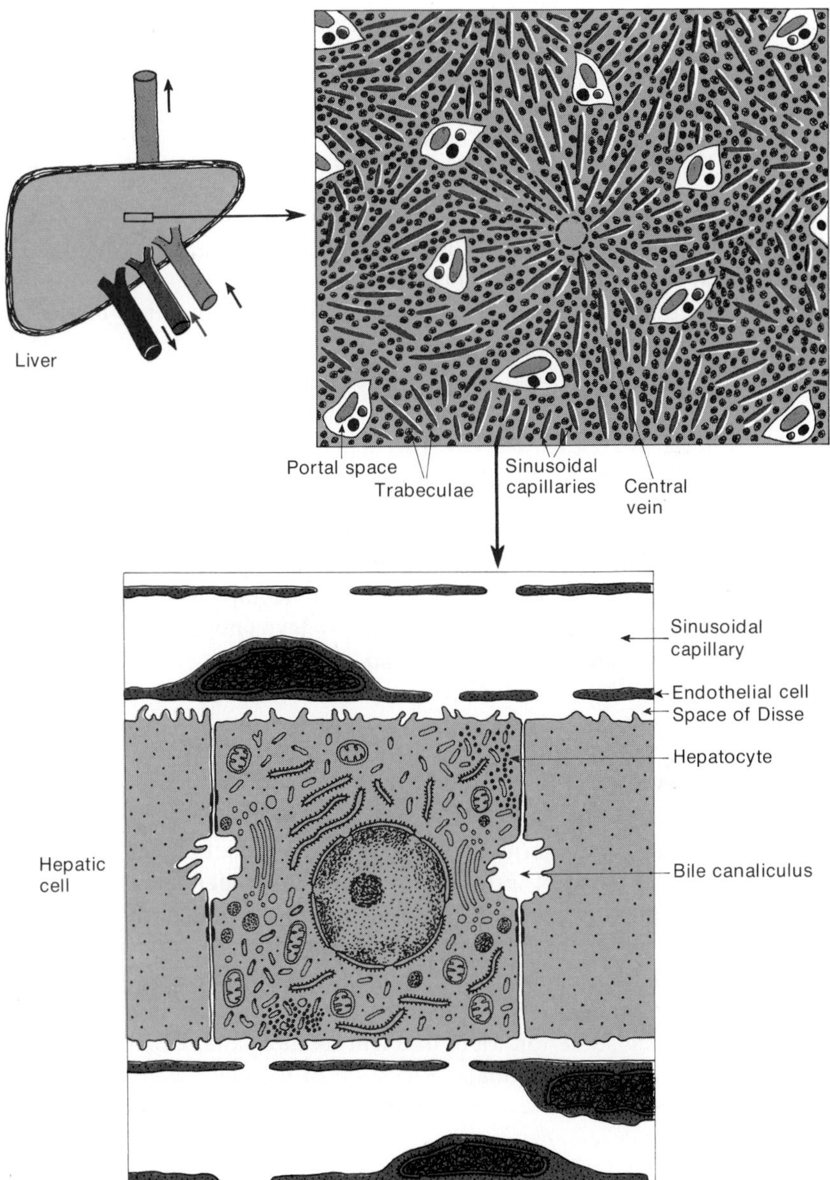

Figure 79. The three structural levels of the liver.

"fiber latticework" of the liver). Some cells bordering the hepatic sinusoids have a macrophagic potential (bordering macrophages). When this potential is activated, the cells hypertrophy, the nucleus enlarges and becomes oval, the nucleolus becomes prominent, and the cytoplasm fills with phagocytized material (red corpuscles, vital stains, India ink, and various particles). These are "Kupffer cells."

D. EXOCRINE PANCREAS

The pancreas is a large exocrine compound acinous gland. Dispersed within are endocrine formations, the islets of Langerhans (see Chapter 19). The glandular parenchyma is divided into *lobules* by layers of connective tissue stemming from the capsule of the organ and containing blood vessels, lymphatics, and nerves.

I. Glandular Acini

The acini of the pancreas are made up of glandular cells with all the morphological characteristics of protein secreting cells, a very abundant granular endoplasmic reticulum, a well-developed supranuclear Golgi apparatus, and, at the apical pole of the cell, an accumulation of secretory granules. The enzymatic content (proteases–trypsinogen, chymotrypsinogen, carboxypolypeptidase–lipase, and amylase) is released into the lumen of the acinus by exocytosis.

II. Excretory Canals

The excretory canals form a system of ramified ducts. Continuing from the acini under the name of intralobular ducts, they later form interlobular ducts, which eventually unite into the collecting ducts. The walls are made up of a simple epithelium (originally cuboidal, then becoming columnar) and are surrounded by a connective tissue layer of progressively increasing thickness. The epithelial cells of these walls elaborate and release into the lumen an aqueous secretion rich in bicarbonates and lacking enzymes. These, together with the enzymatic secretion of the acini, contribute to the formation of "pancreatic juice" that is released into the duodenum.

16

Urinary System

A. GENERAL STRUCTURE

I. Kidney

When examined with the naked eye or a magnifying glass, three principal portions can be distinguished in a median sagittal section of the kid-

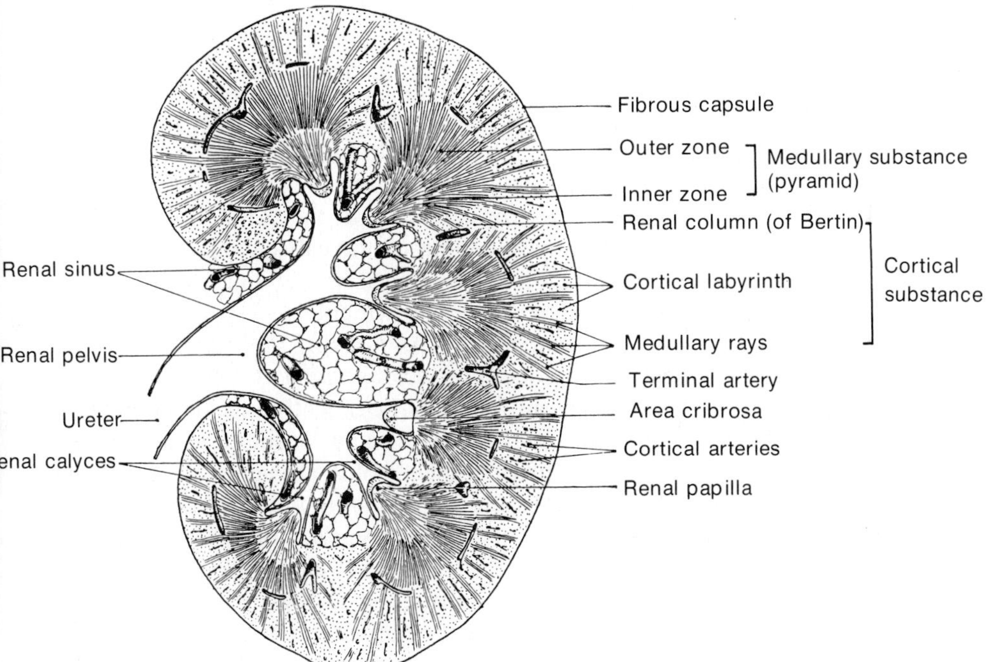

Figure 80. Schematic representation of a section of a kidney. (After O. Bucher, 1973.)

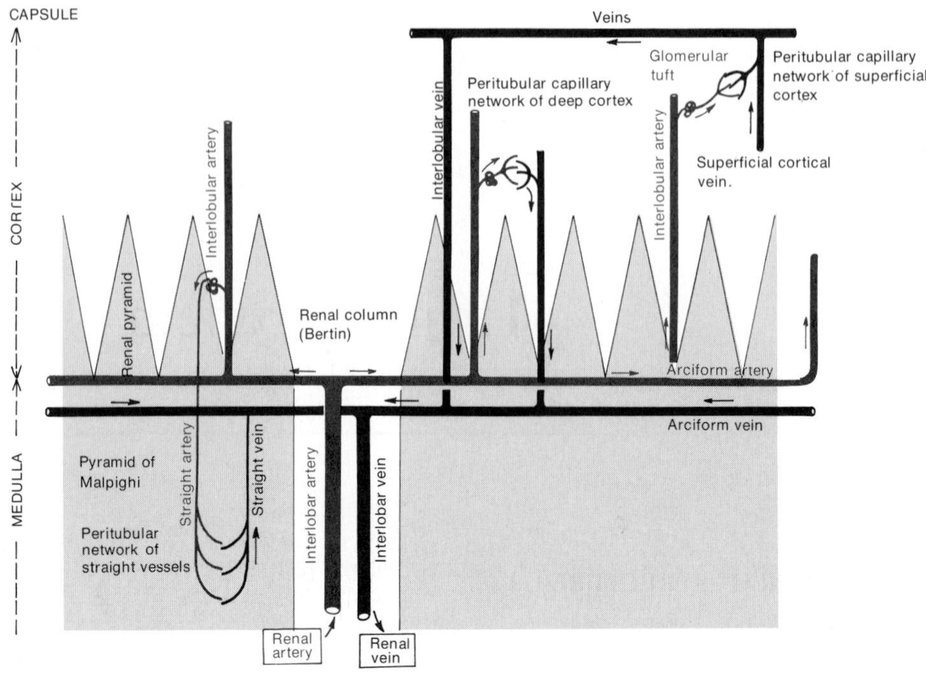

Figure 81. Renal vascularization.

ney. The periphery of the organ is surrounded by a capsule, continuous with the connective tissue of the hilum, which surrounds the calyces and the pelvis. The inner zone or medulla consists of about 8 to 18 renal pyramids whose apices are perforated by openings of the uriniferous tubules. Each apex protrudes into a corresponding minor calyx while the base of the pyramid abuts against the cortex. Cortical tissue capping pyramidal tissue is clearly distinguished by its reddish-brown color.

Medulla and cortex are made up of portions of the nephrons of the kidney. With the optical microscope, the various segments of the nephrons are observed to be covered by an interstitial connective tissue containing numerous blood vessels, some lymphatics, and vasomotor autonomic nerves. The lobar arteries, which are branches of the renal artery, enter the cortical columns (of Bertin) and reach the base of the renal pyramids, splitting into arcuate arteries that do not anastomose with others. Interlobular arteries branch off from the arcuate arteries and run perpendicular to the surface of the kidney. From interlobular arteries spring afferent glomerular arterioles, which terminate in loops of glomerular capillaries. Blood exits

TABLE 27. Histology of the Urinary Ducts

Urinary Ducts		Mucosa: Epithelium	Mucosa: Lamina Propria	Muscularis	Adventitia
Calyces		Transitional	Vascular connective tissue without glands	Two layers of smooth muscle cells: inner longitudinal and outer circular (+ a third, outer longitudinal layer, in the lower third of the ureter)	Connective tissue
Cortex					
Ureter					
Bladder				Plexiform (with a smooth sphincter at the entrance of the ureter)	Replaced partially by the peritoneal serosa
Urethra	Male	Pseudostratified columnar ↓ Stratified columnar ↓ Nonkeratinized stratified squamous with intra-epithelial mucous glands	Surrounded by the prostate ↓ Surrounded by the striated muscles of the perineum ↓ Surrounded by the spongy body of the penis (+ extra-epithelial glands)	Two layers of smooth muscle cells: inner longitudinal and outer circular (except at the level of the spongy ureter)	
	Female	Transitional Stratified columnar Nonkeratinized stratified squamous, with intra-epithelial mucous glands	Connective tissue with extraepithelial glands	Two layers of smooth muscle cells: inner longitudinal and outer circular	Connective tissue

via efferent glomerular arterioles, which give rise to the peritubular capillary network.

Efferent glomerular arterioles of juxtamedullary nephrons branch into descending straight arteries which supply the medulla.* Blood from the peritubular capillary networks of the cortex and medullary capillary networks deriving from the straight arteries is returned to venules and veins whose course is comparable to that of the arterial vessels (interlobular veins and straight veins, arcuate veins, interlobar veins, and renal vein).

II. Urinary Ducts (see Table 27)

B. THE NEPHRON

Urine formation takes place in the nephrons (of which there are about 1,000,000 in each kidney) and consists of two main stages: ultrafiltration of the blood plasma in the glomerulus, and reabsorption and/or secretion of certain substances in the tubule.

I. Filtration Level: The Glomerulus

Capillary Tuft

The *afferent* glomerular artery at the vascular pole of the glomerulus divides into five or six arterioles, from which spring about 20 capillary loops. These terminate in the *efferent* glomerular artery, which exits the glomerulus at the vascular pole. Capillary loops consist of three elements:

*Some straight medullary arteries spring directly from the arcuate arteries and interlobular arteries.

TABLE 28. Segments of the Nephron

Nephron	Glomerulus	
	Tubule	*Proximal Tubule:* Proximal convoluted tubule Large descending branch of loop of Henle
		Small Loop of Henle: Small descending branch of loop of Henle Small ascending branch of loop of Henle
		Distal Tubule: Large ascending branch of loop of Henle Distal convoluted tubule Uniting canal
		Collecting Tubule: Ending in the papillary canal opening at the apex of the pyramids of Malpighi

endothelial cells of the capillaries, a *basal lamina,* and adjacent *mesangial cells.* The flattened and interdigitated simple squamous endothelial cells of the capillaries are pierced by pores occasionally supplied with a diaphragm. The basal lamina is continuous with that of the endothelium of the afferent and efferent arteries of the glomerulus, and is *uninterrupted.* It surrounds the capillary endothelium, but has the special characteristic of forming (in the capillary loop) a "mesentery-like" structure with its two layers becoming fused together. Mesangial cells, enveloped by this "mesentery," rest between the endothelial cells of adjacent capillaries (hence the term *mesangial*—"between vessels").

The Filtration Cavity

This cavity is bounded by Bowman's capsule, a parietal and visceral layer of epithelium. The parietal layer of simple squamous epithelium facing the lumen rests on a basal lamina. The visceral layer, continuous with the parietal layer at the vascular pole, is made of a discontinuous layer of cells called *podocytes.* Podocytes have numerous cytoplasmic processes, which in turn give rise to a multitude of smaller processes ("pedicels of the podocytes"), which interdigitate and attach to the outer surface of the basal lamina of the capillaries.

Filtration Barrier

The glomerular filtrate is the result of plasma ultrafiltration through a barrier consisting of (1) fenestrated capillary endothelium, allowing passage

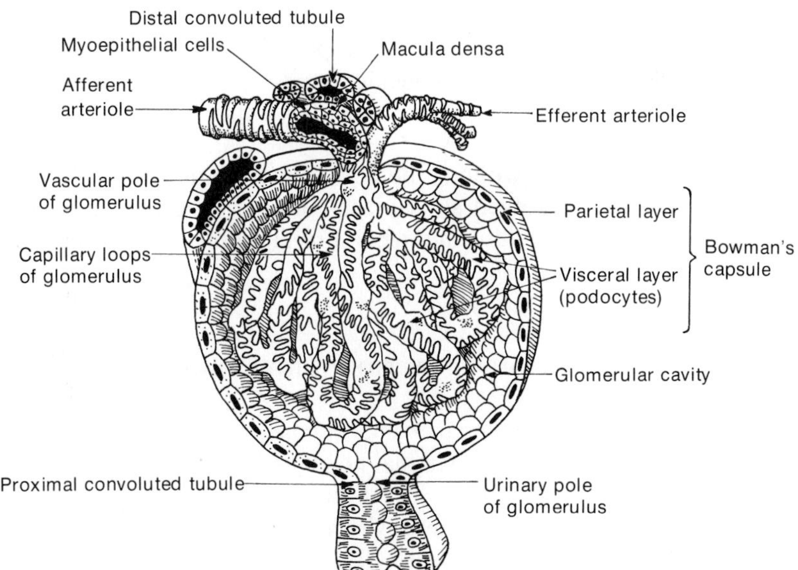

Figure 82. Three-dimensional, schematic representation of a glomerulus of Malpighi. (Redrawn after W. Bloom and D. W. Fawcett, 1975.)

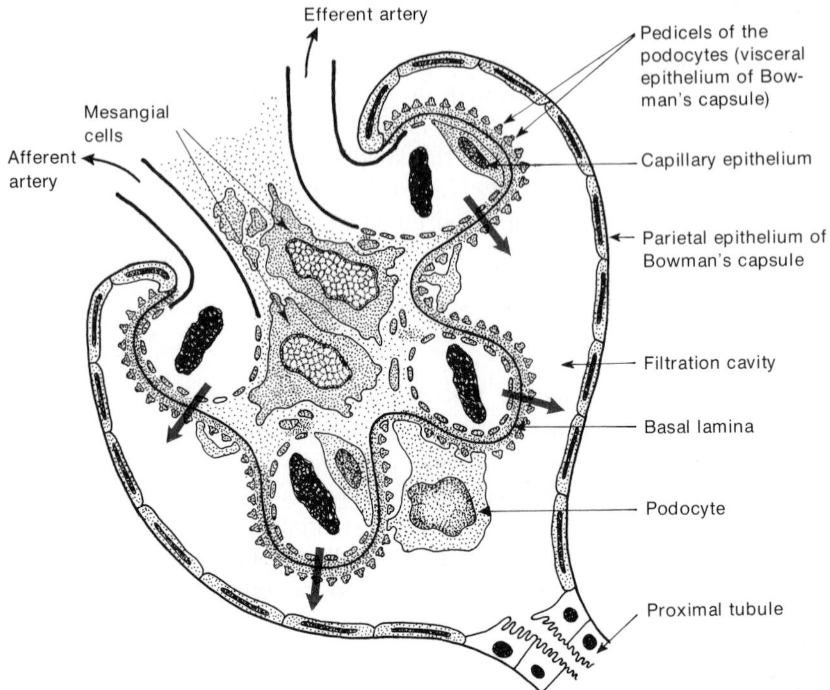

Figure 83. Schematic diagram of the renal glomerulus. (Redrawn after S. L. Galbraith, 1971.)

by diffusion and/or through the pores, (2) capillary basal lamina, preventing the passage only of very large molecules, and (3) most importantly, the membrane uniting the pedicels of the podocytes, a fine sieve preventing the passage of smaller molecules.

Passive ultrafiltration, without the active intervention of cells, allows the passage of water, dissolved substances (glucose, uric acid, urea, creatinine, phosphates, electrolytes), and small protein molecules with a molecular weight of less than 70,000.

II. Site of Reabsorption–Secretion: The Tubule

a. Proximal Tubule. The proximal tubule, formed of simple columnar epithelium resting on a basal lamina, consists of cells characterized by: (1) elongated microvilli forming a "brush border" at the apical poles; (2) deep folds in the basal membrane into which cytoplasmic processes extend to interdigitate with those of adjacent cells; (3) elongated mitochondria arranged perpendicularly to the membrane of the basal pole and between

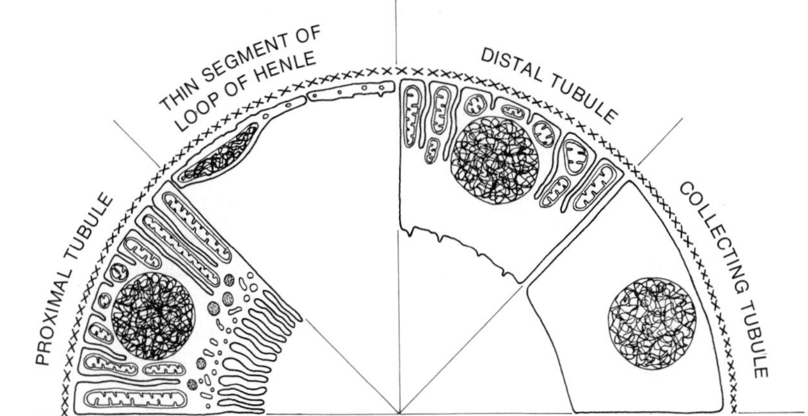

Figure 84. Schematic diagram of the epithelium of the renal tubule, as seen with the electron microscope.

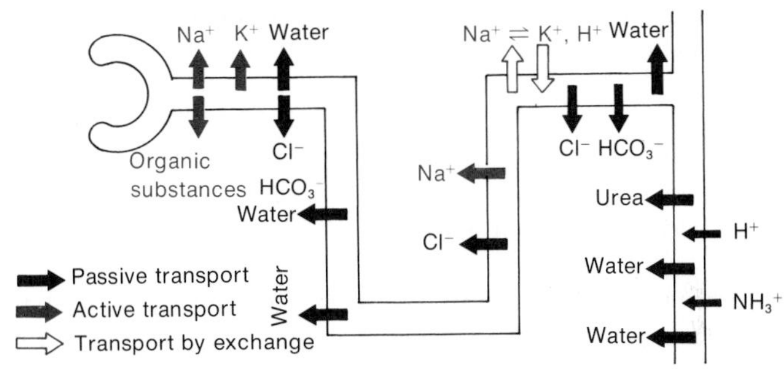

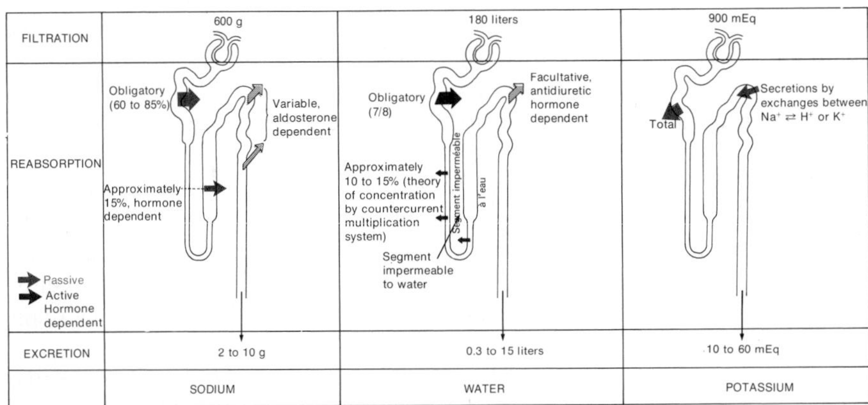

Figure 85. Hydrolytic exchanges in the nephron. (Redrawn after M. Legrain: Traite de Biologie Clinique. Paris, Maloine, 1971.)

membrane folds; and (4) vesicles, vacuoles, and lysosomes in the apical cytoplasm.

b. Thin Loop of Henle. The thin loop of Henle has a small diameter, about the size of a capillary. Its wall is made of simple squamous epithelium resting on a basal lamina.

c. Distal Tubule. The distal tubule is composed of simple cuboidal epithelium resting on a basal lamina. The cells are characterized by short, stubby microvilli at the apical poles, deep infoldings of the membrane of its basal pole, with cytoplasmic processes similar to those of the proximal tubule, and elongated mitochondria located between membrane infoldings.

d. Collecting Tubule. The collecting tubule consists of simple cuboidal or columnar epithelium resting on its basal lamina.

Over all its length, the tubular epithelium is the site of active and/or passive exchanges between the tubular lumen and the peritubular capillary network. The relationship between the structure of the various segments of the tubule and the fundamental physiological events taking place, is poorly understood. It has been well established, however, that (1) the epithelium of the proximal tubule presents structures reflecting an intense reabsorptive activity, and (2) the thin layer of epithelium of the loop of Henle, with its abundant pinocytotic vesicles, indicates important movements of water and electrolytes (via the countercurrent multiplication system).

III. Short and Long Nephrons

Nephrons with a glomerulus in the superficial (outer) cortical region have a small glomerulus (hence a smaller filtration surface) and a short thin loop of Henle, which does not descend beyond the outer medulla. Efferent arterioles form the peritubular capillary network prior to rejoining the superficial cortical veins. In humans, these nephrons with short loops make up about 80 to 90 per cent of the nephron. They have a small sodium reabsorption capacity ("salt-losing nephrons").

Nephrons with a glomerulus located in the deep juxtamedullary area of the cortex have a large glomerulus (hence a large filtration surface) and a long thin loop of Henle descending into the inner medulla. Efferent arterioles have a dual destination: some form the deep peritubular capillary networks, which rejoin the interlobular veins, and others form straight vessels which, after a long path through the medulla, rejoin the arcuate veins. They have a great sodium reabsorption capacity ("salt-retaining nephrons").

Homeostasis is maintained by: (1) the degree of activity of these two types of nephrons under the influence of the sympathetic nervous system, (2) the rate of circulating catecholamines, and (3) the renin-angiotensin system (see *Juxtaglomerular apparatus).*

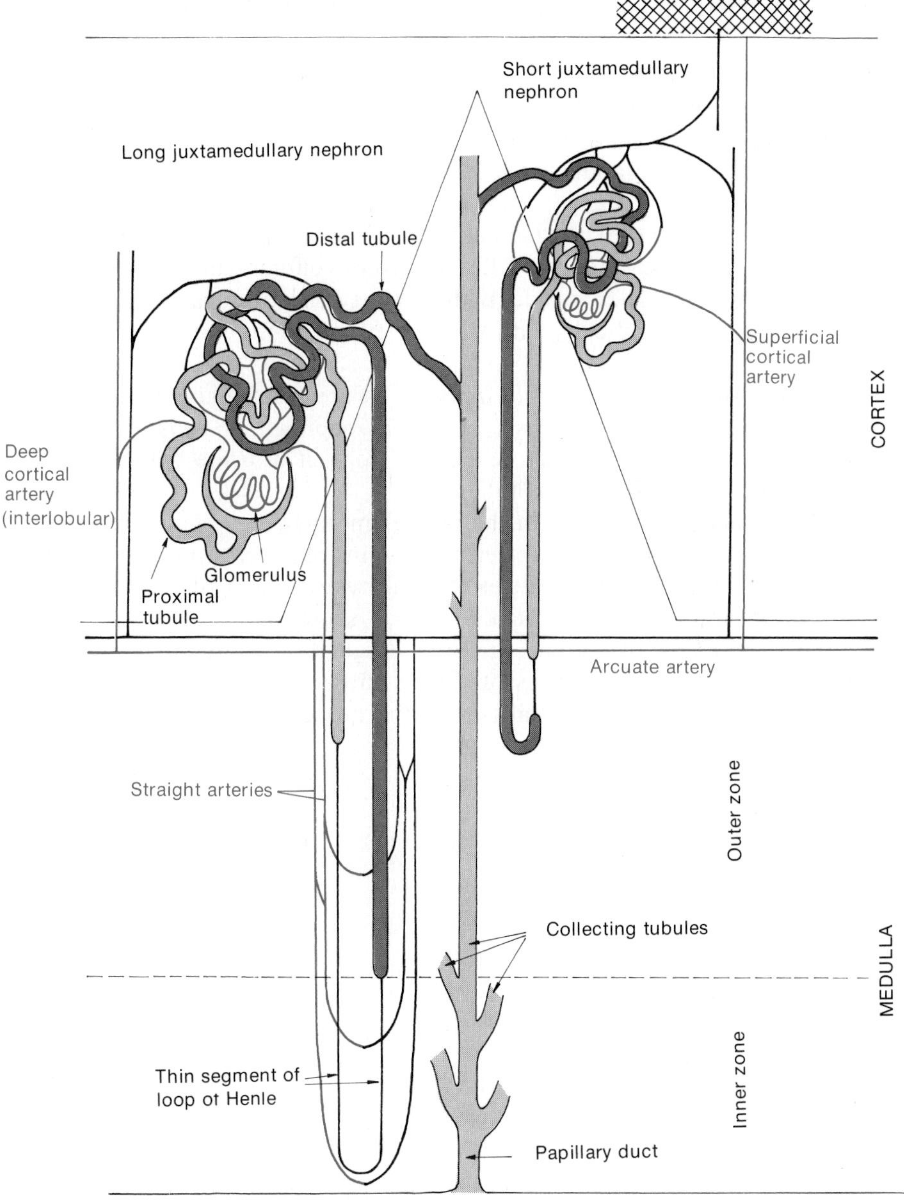

Figure 86. Schematic representation of a nephron.

IV. Juxtaglomerular Apparatus

The juxtaglomerular apparatus, located in the angle formed by afferent and efferent glomerular arteries, consists of myoepithelioid (juxtaglomerular) cells, reticular (lacis) cells, and the macula densa.

Juxtaglomerular Cells. *Juxtaglomerular cells* appear to be highly modified smooth muscle cells in the wall of the afferent artery at the point where it penetrates the glomerulus. These "myoepithelioid cells" are separated from the endothelium of the afferent artery only by a simple basal lamina. Their cytoplasm is characterized by the presence of myofibrils and endocrine secretory granules. These are the cells that secrete renin.

Lacis Cells. *Lacis cells* (sometimes called extraglomerular mesangial cells) are located between the afferent artery, efferent artery, and distal convoluted tubule. They reside within a network of basal laminae, and resemble the mesangial cells with which they are continuous.

Macula Densa. The *macula densa* is an area of the convoluted distal tubule whose basal lamina rests on the myoepithelioid cells. The intercellular spaces at this level allow a direct contact of urine with the basal lamina of the distal convoluted tubule.

The myoepithelioid cells of the juxtaglomerular complex secrete renin into the blood of the afferent arteriole. Renin transforms angiotensinogen into angiotensin. The latter causes arterial hypertension (mainly by vasoconstriction and stimulation of aldosterone secretion), and therefore decreased elimination of sodium in urine. Regulation of renin secretion is linked to the level of blood pressure in the afferent arteriole and to the rate of sodium retention in the distal tubule (the macula densa playing the role of osmoreceptor).

17

Male Reproductive System

The male reproductive system consists of two gonads *(testes),* genital ducts *(efferent ducts, ductus epididymidis, ductus deferens, ejaculatory ducts,* and *urethra),* associated endocrine glands *(interstitial cells),* and exocrine glands *(seminiferous tubules, seminal vesicles, prostate,* and *bulbourethral glands).*

The *testes* (see Fig. 91) are bilateral structures located outside the body cavity in the *scrotum.* A double layer of pinched-off peritoneum, the *tunica vaginalis,* covers the testis, except at the hilum. The *tunica albuginea,* which is a thick, firm capsule of white fibrous connective tissue, invests the entire bean-shaped testis. The testis is subdivided into 250 compartments by connective tissue extensions of the capsule converging at the hilum. Within each compartment are located two to four highly coiled *seminiferous tubules* in a bed of loose areolar vascular connective tissue. The endocrine cells of the testis *(interstitial cells)* are scattered throughout the loose connective tissue in the compartment, forming a diffuse endocrine gland.

The seminiferous tubules straighten out in the hilum as the *tubuli recti,* form a network (the *rete testes*), and exit as 12 efferent ducts.

A. SECRETION OF ANDROGEN HORMONES

The secretion of the testicular androgenic hormone, testosterone, is carried out by endocrine glandular cells scattered throughout the reticular connective tissue of the testes (Leydig cells or interstitial cells of the testis). These cells present the same morphological characteristics as steroid secreting cells.* Their activity is dependent on the pituitary hormone LH/ICSH (interstitial cell stimulating hormone).

B. ELABORATION OF SPERM

I. Formation of Spermatozoa in the Seminiferous Tubules of the Testes

The walls of the seminiferous tubules in the vascular connective tissue stroma of the testicular lobules consist of germinal cells and supporting cells (Sertoli).

*They are peculiar in containing cytoplasmic protein formations with a crystalline nature (crystals of Reinke), whose role is unknown.

Cells of Germinal Lineage

a. Spermatogonia. Spermatogonia are large, rounded cells with a large nucleus (with a diploid number of 46 chromosomes), located at the periphery of the tubules, against their basal lamina. Each spermatogonium, in about 74 days, will give rise to 16 spermatozoa.

b. Primary Spermatocytes. The primary spermatocytes, which have 2n or 46 chromosomes arise from spermatogonia by normal mitosis and undergo a first meiotic division, giving rise to secondary spermatocytes. The prophase of this division (comprising leptotene, zygotene, pachytene, and diplotene) is very long, permitting visualization of many primary spermatocytes in sections of seminiferous tubules.

c. Secondary Spermatocytes. Secondary spermatocytes (23 chromosomes) are small and quickly undergo a second meiotic division, producing the spermatids. Therefore, they are rarely visible in sections.

d. Spermatids. The spermatids (23 chromosomes) are small, slightly elongated cells. They are haploid and no longer divide but become transformed into spermatozoa through the following changes: elongation of the nucleus, which becomes fusiform; formation of an acrosome at the Golgi complex; migration of centrioles; formation of a flagellum from the distal centriole; regrouping of the mitochondria around the base of the flagellum; and decrease in cytoplasm.

e. Spermatozoa. The spermatozoa consist of a head, a neck, and a tail.

1. The *head* contains a fusiform nucleus (with 23 chromosomes), with the acrosome capping its anterior pole.
2. The *neck,* which is short and shrivelled, contains a proximal centriole and a distal centriole (which gives rise to the flagellum).
3. The *tail* consists of *(a) the middle piece,* somewhat distended, made up of a fibrous axial complex (nine pairs of peripheral tubules and one pair of central tubules), surrounded by a sheath of mitochondria arranged regularly in a spiral; *(b)* the *principal piece,* about five times longer than the head, neck, and middle piece combined, containing the continuation of the axial fibrous complex of the flagellum, surrounded by a fibrous sheath; and *(c)* the *end piece,* which is the very short termination of the flagellum.

Supporting (Sertoli) Cells

These cells extend from the periphery of the lumen of the seminiferous tubules, and between them are scattered germinal cells in various stages. This arrangement clearly shows the important role the Sertoli cells play in the sequence of events during spermatogenesis—protection and nutrition of germinal cells and release of mature spermatozoa into the lumen of the seminiferous tubules.

Leydig cells
Capillary
Connective tissue
Spermatogonium
Spermatocyte I
Nucleus of
Sertoli cell
Spermatid
Spermatocyte II
Spermatozoon
Seminiferous tubule

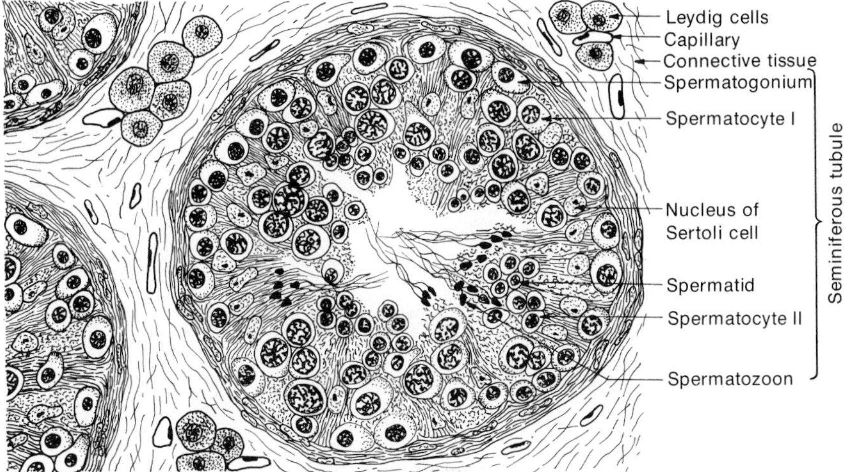

Figure 87. Testes (light microscope, ×500). (Modified after O. Bucher, 1973.)

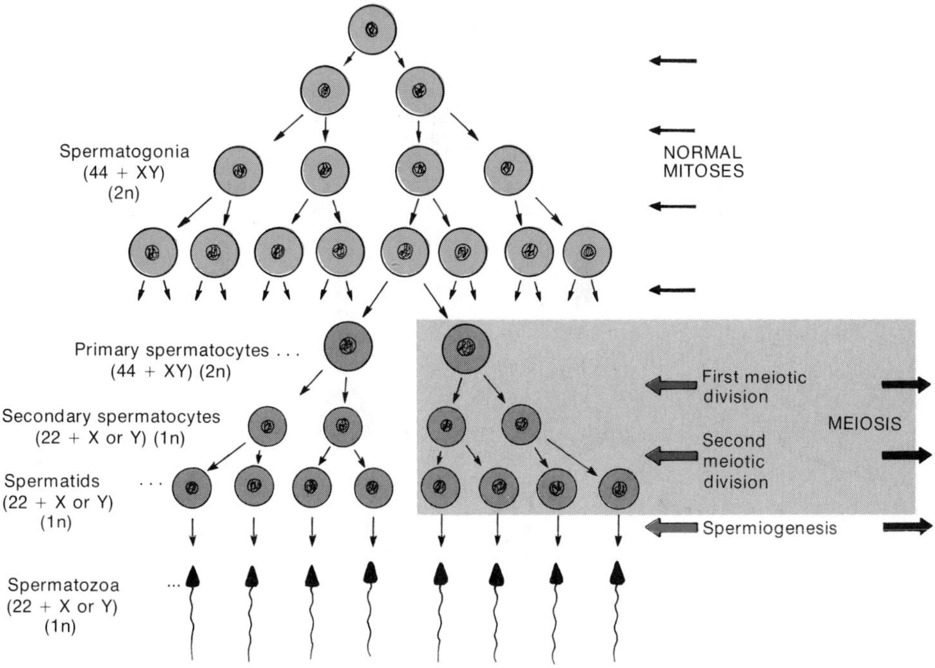

Spermatogonia
(44 + XY)
(2n)
NORMAL
MITOSES
Primary spermatocytes . . .
(44 + XY) (2n)
Secondary spermatocytes
(22 + X or Y) (1n)
Spermatids . . .
(22 + X or Y)
(1n)
Spermatozoa . . .
(22 + X or Y)
(1n)
First meiotic
division
Second
meiotic
division
MEIOSIS
Spermiogenesis

Figure 88. Diagram of the formation of spermatozoa in the seminiferous tubules of the testes (spermatogenesis).

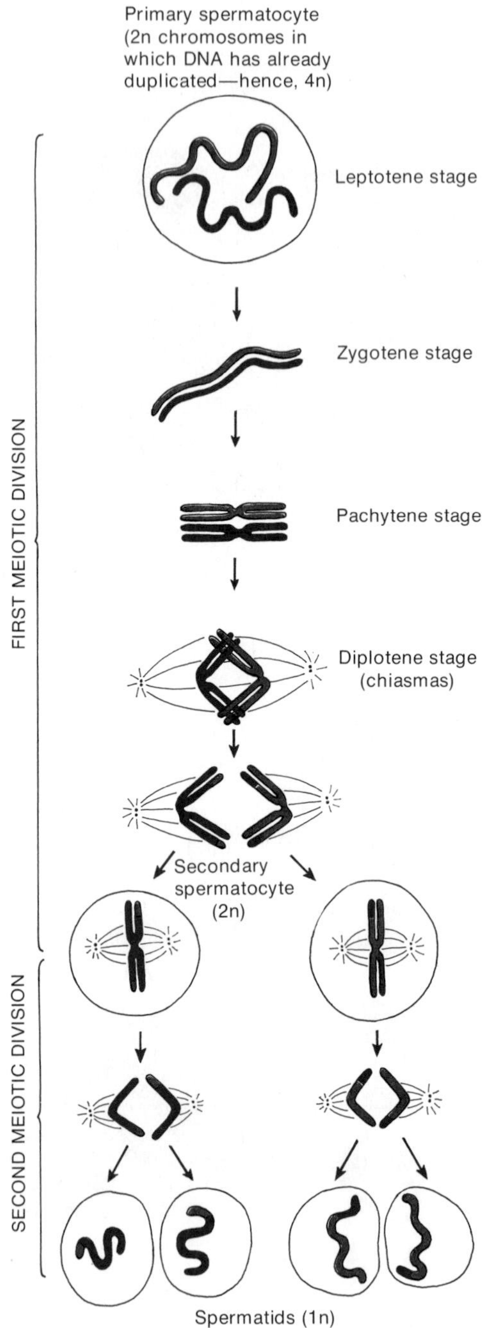

Figure 89. Schematic representation of the principal stages of meiosis. (Only one pair of homologous chromosomes has been represented.) It can be seen that one initial DNA replication takes place for each two successive cell divisions, so that one cell with 2n chromosomes finally gives rise to four cells with 1n chromosomes.

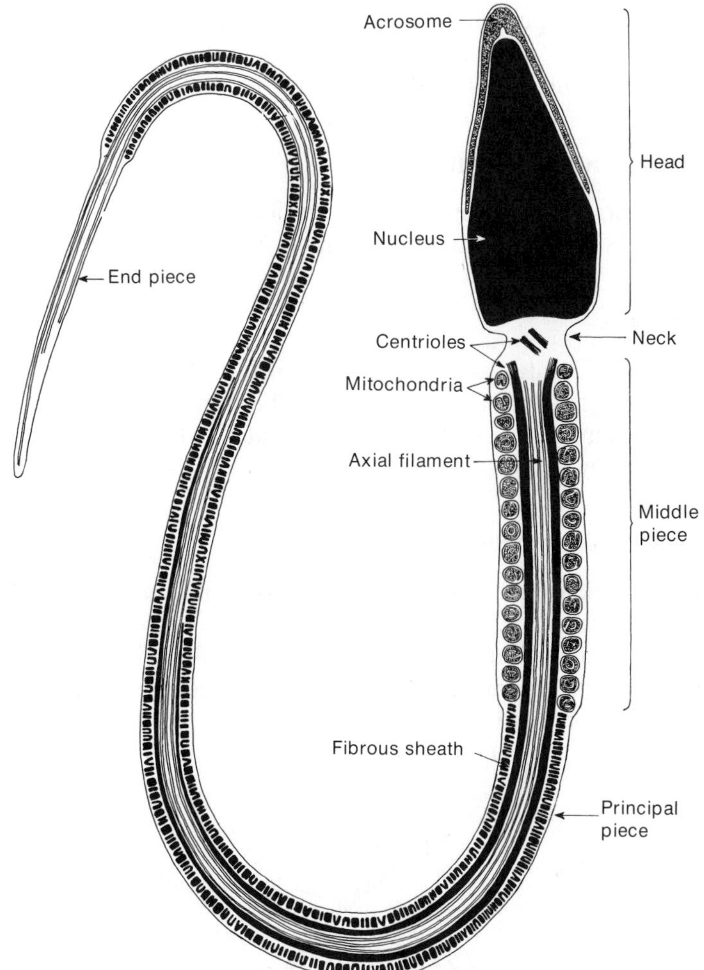

Figure 90. Schematic representation of the ultrastructure of a spermatozoon. (Modified after T. L. Lentz.)

II. Conduction of Spermatozoa and Secretion of Seminal Fluid

Once the spermatozoa are formed inside the seminiferous tubules of the testes, they are conveyed toward the tubuli recti and rete testis, and later to the extratesticular ducts (efferent ducts, epididymal duct, ductus deferens, ejaculatory duct, and urethra). Along this course, the epithelium of certain parts of the spermatic ducts (especially epididymis) and of certain glands (i.e., seminal vesicles, prostate, and bulbourethral glands of Cowper) secretes a seminal fluid in which the spermatozoa swim freely.

Tubuli Recti and Rete Testis

These converge at the hilum, joining seminiferous tubules and efferent ducts. Their walls consist of simple squamous epithelium.

Efferent Ducts

The ductuli efferentes are highly coiled inside the efferent (vascular) cones to form the head of the epididymis. The lumen is lined by simple columnar epithelium with ciliated cells, glandular cells, and replacement cells, surrounded by some smooth muscle cells.

The Ductus Epididymidis

The ductus epididymidis follows a tortuous, coiled course, and forms, together with the vascularized connective tissue, the body and head of the epididymis. Its regular lumen is bordered by a simple epithelium made of replacement cells and columnar cells. The latter possess stereocilia at their apical poles, and secretion granules and lysosomes are found in the cytoplasm. This duct is surrounded by a thin layer of smooth muscle cells. In

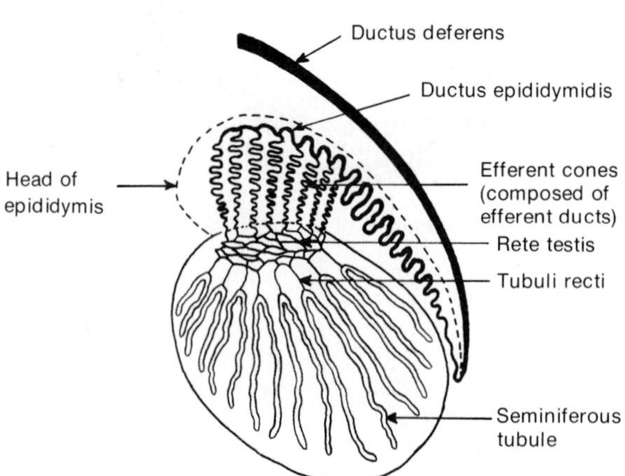

Figure 91. Spermatic ducts. (Modified after A. Giroud and A. Lelievre, 1969.)

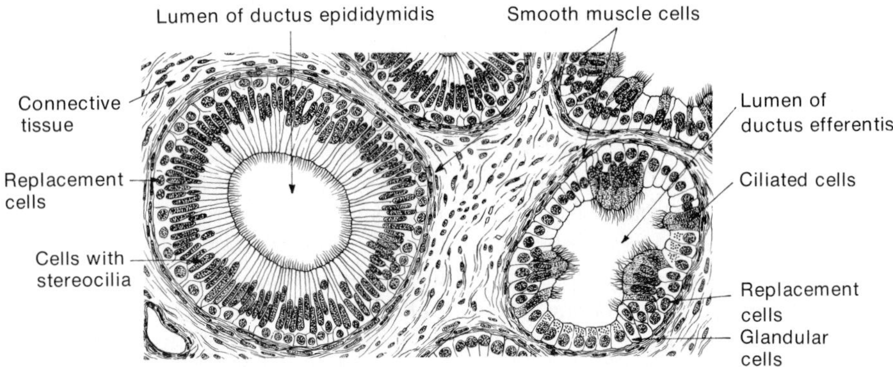

Figure 92. Schematic representation of a section of epididymis as seen with the light microscope. *Left,* a section of the ductus epididymidis; *right,* a section of the efferent duct (×250). (After W. Bargmann, 1967.)

addition to conveying sperm through contractions of its smooth musculature, the ductus epididymidis plays an absorptive role (stereocilia, lysosomes) and a secretory role (granules of secretion).

"Secretions of epididymal cells have a triple function: they maintain vitality of spermatozoa; enhance the motility inherent to spermatozoa; and render spermatozoa unfit for fecundation through decapacitation" (Girod and Czyba, 1972).

Ductus Deferens

The wall of the ductus deferens, which is thick compared to the diameter of its lumen, consists of three concentric layers. The mucosa has an epithelium similar to that of the ductus epididymidis, and a lamina propria of loose connective tissue. The muscularis is very thick and the adventitia contains numerous vessels and nerves. Its terminal portion thickens into a

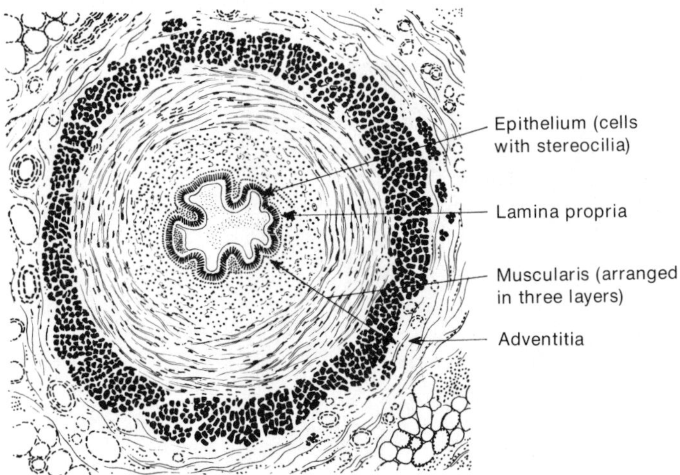

Figure 93. Schematic representation of a section of the ductus deferens as seen with the light microscope (×40). (After W. Bargmann, 1967.)

bulb, the "ampulla," which may serve as a reservoir for sperm between ejaculations.

Seminal Vesicles

The mucosa forms numerous folds and consists of a simple columnar epithelium made up of glandular cells which secrete a light and viscid liquid (containing ascorbic acid, fructose–which is an essential metabolite for the spermatozoa–citric acid, phosphorylcholine, and prostaglandin). A loose connective tissue lamina propria, a thin muscularis, and an adventitia containing numerous vessels and nerves make up the rest of the wall.

Together with the distal extremity of the ductus deferens (forming a sort of diverticulum) they make up the ejaculatory ducts.

Ejaculatory Ducts

The epithelium of the ejaculatory ducts is simple columnar with no notable differentiation. It is demarcated from the prostatic stroma by a thin layer of smooth connective tissue.

Urethra

The urethra consists of three areas with different structural characteristics: pars prostatica, pars membranacea, and pars spongiosa (see Chapter 16, *Urinary System*).

Prostate

The prostate is composed of about 50 tubulo-alveolar glandular lobules, from which about 20 excretory ducts open into the prostatic urethra, which traverses it. The glandular epithelium is simple columnar or cuboidal, with rounded basal nuclei and apical secretory granules. Lamellar protein concretions can be seen in the lumen of the glands. The dense connective tissue located between the glandular elements contains smooth muscle

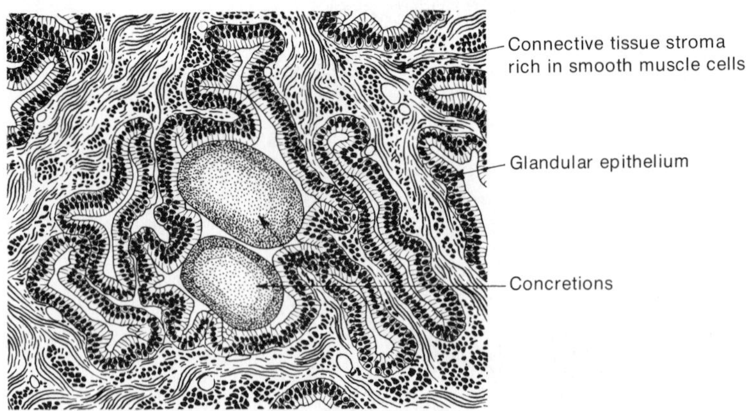

Figure 94. Schematic representation of a section of prostate as seen with the light microscope (×150). (After W. Bargmann, 1967.)

cells in great number, plus capillaries and nerves. The secretory fluid is rich in amino acids, citric acids, and enzymes (especially alkaline and acid phosphatase).

Bulbourethral Glands (of Cowper)

These are compound, tubulo-alveolar mucous glands which release their secretory product into pars spongiosa of the urethra.

III. Semen

Semen, which is discharged during ejaculation (2 to 5 ml. per ejaculation) consists of spermatozoa suspended in the seminal fluid.

Spermatozoa

Normally there are 60,000 to 100,000 spermatozoa per $mm.^3$ In an average ejaculate, 10 to 20 per cent of spermatozoa are found to be morphologically abnormal. Under normal circumstances, in sperm examined less than two hours after ejaculation, about 80 per cent of the spermatozoa are motile. Twenty-four hours after ejaculation, only 15 per cent retain normal motility. This motility is a very important functional characteristic of the spermatozoa, and its inhibition (by certain chemical agents) completely destroys fertilizing capacity. When sperm is conserved at low temperatures, its vitality is preserved and it retains its fertilizing capacities. To become capable of fertilizing an ovum, spermatozoa undergo a "capacitation" on coming into contact with the uterine and tubal mucosae.

Seminal Fluid

The seminal fluid contains water, mineral salts, proteins, free amino acids, spermine, choline, fructose, and prostaglandins.

C. THE SEX ACT

The sex act, leading to ejaculation of semen, comprises three successive phenomena: erection, ejaculation, and detumescence.

I. Erection

The corpora spongiosa (traversed by the penile urethra) and the two corpora cavernosa of the penis are made of erectile tissue. The three bodies are surrounded by a dense fibroelastic tunica albuginea. Arteries and veins contain, in most of the cases, "sphincters" made of smooth muscle cells. Under the influence of erotic stimulations via medullary reflex arcs, smooth muscle cells of arterial sphincters relax and blood flows freely into the erectile tissue. Filling of spaces is accompanied by the compression of the peripheral venous plexuses. This restriction of venous drainage (increased by contraction of venous sphincters) further slows down circulation and dilates the spaces, causing a tumescence of the corpora spongiosa and cavernosa. The concomitant erectness of the penis is linked to the contraction of smooth muscle cells of the erectile tissue and striated muscles of the anterior perineum.

II. Ejaculation

Ejaculation is preceded by the accumulation of sperm in the urethra above the striated muscle sphincter which, owing to its tonus, prevents outflow. Ejaculation is initiated by spasmodic reflex contractions of perineal muscles acting upon the urethral sphincter and allowing the release of sperm.

III. Detumescence

After ejaculation, the smooth muscle cells of the arterial blockage devices contract, thus stopping blood flow in the spaces of the erectile tissue. The smooth muscle cells of the erectile tissue relax, as do the venous sphincters, and venous drainage is restored, leading to progressive detumescence of the penis.

18

Female Reproductive System

The female reproductive system consists of two gonads (ovaries), the genital ducts (two oviducts, the uterus, and the vagina), and the external genitalia (vulva). The structure of these organs and accessories undergoes very important modifications in the various stages of genital life (puberty, pregnancy, menopause), and also shows cyclic variations depending on hormonal interrelationships between the hypothalamus-hypophysis and ovary during the period of genital activity.

A. BASIC STRUCTURES

I. Ovary

The ovary is surrounded by simple cuboidal epithelium continuous with peritoneal mesothelium of the mesovarium. The ovary consists of two zones.

1. *A thick cortical zone,* situated at the periphery, contains the ovarian follicles dispersed throughout the ovarian stroma. Stromal connective tissue condenses beneath the surface epithelium forming a dense fibrous layer, the *albuginea.*

2. *A medullary zone,* located centrally with loose connective tissue, contains numerous blood and lymph vessels and nerves.

TABLE 29. Histology of the Female Reproductive Tract

		Oviducts	Uterus: Fundus and Body	Uterus: Cervix, Inner	Uterus: Cervix, Outer	Vagina
MUCOSA	Epithelium	Simple columnar with ciliated cells (predominant) and secretory cells	Simple columnar with ciliated cells and secretory cells (mucus and polysaccharides)		Nonkeratinized stratified squamous (cells rich in glycogen)	
MUCOSA	Lamina Propria: *Connective Tissue*	Rich in cells, and in blood and lymph vessels	Irregular stellate cells; reticular fibers; ground substance rich in mucopolysaccharides; numerous blood and lymph vessels	Dense		Rich in: elastic fibers; lymphoid cells; blood vessels (venous plexus and lymphatics)
MUCOSA	Lamina Propria: *Glands*		Simple tubular exocrine glands made up of columnar cells identical to those of the epithelium	"Cervical" glands, tubulo-alveolar, ramified, pure mucosal		
MUSCULARIS		Two layers of smooth muscle cells: inner circular and outer longitudinal	Fascicles of smooth muscle cells arranged in three layers: inner layer, predominantly longitudinal; thick middle layer, predominantly circular and oblique; outer layer, predominantly longitudinal	Fascicles of smooth muscle cells, predominantly circular		Fascicles of smooth muscle cells, circular and especially longitudinal (+ striated muscles of the perineum surrounding the vagina)
SEROSA OR ADVENTITIA		Thick, loose, peritoneal serosa continuous with the mesosalpinx; rich in adipose cells, vessels, and nerves	Peritoneal serosa of the fundus of the posterior face of the body			Adventitia containing vessels and nerves, in the rectouterine fossa replaced by the peritoneal serosa ("pouch of Douglas")

TABLE 29. ***(Continued)***

VULVA (EXTERNAL GENITAL ORGANS)	*Labia Majora*	Skin folds containing sweat glands, sebaceous glands, and hairs (numerous and thick at the outside, scarce and thin at the inside)	SENSORY ZONES (NUMEROUS NERVE ENDINGS: CORPUSCLES OF MEISSNER, GENITAL CORPUSCLES, CORPUSCLES OF PACINI)
	Labia Minora	Slightly dekeratinized skin folds, containing sweat glands and sebaceous glands, but no hairs	
	Clitoris	Rudimentary erectile organ made of erectile tissue covered by an epithelium identical to that of the vestibule	
	Vestibule	Covered by mucosa of nonkeratinized stratified squamous epithelium; opening into it is the uterine meatus (the vaginal orifice that is incompletely closed in the virgin by the hymen) and the excreting tubules of the glands of Bartholin	
	Glands of Bartholin	Mucous glands located in the lateral walls of the vestibule on each side of the vagina	

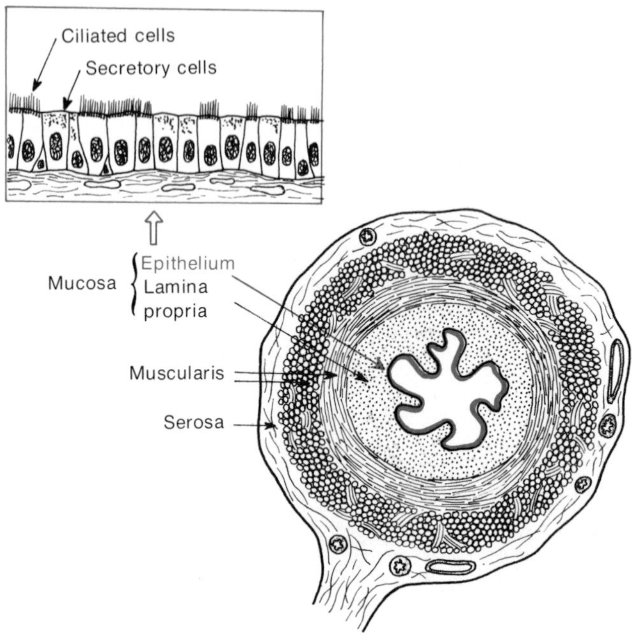

Figure 95. Schematic representation of a section of the fallopian (uterine) tube.

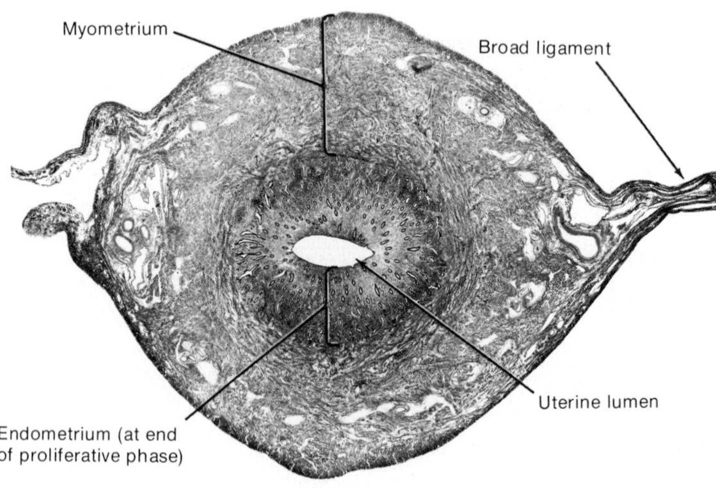

Figure 96. Uterus in transverse section. (After H. Mizoguchi, in W. Bloom and D. W. Fawcett, 1975.)

II. Genital Ducts and External Genital Organs

III. The Breasts

The mammary gland is a compound tubulo-alveolar exocrine gland made of 15 to 20 lobes, subdivided into lobules. In its structure it is schematically the same as other compound exocrine glands. There is a system of excretory ducts, which ramify successively into intralobular, interlobular, and finally interlobar ducts (the primary ducts that open at the nipple); tubulo-alveolar secretory portions surrounded by myoepithelial cells at the ends of the interlobular ducts; and enveloping connective tissue, containing the blood and lymph vessels.

B. BEFORE PUBERTY

At birth, the ovaries contain approximately 400,000 primordial oocytes (arrested during the prophase stage of the first meiotic division) surrounded by a layer of flattened follicular cells. The absence of hypothalamo-hypophyseal stimulation between birth and puberty explains why these primordial follicles do not mature and why many degenerate (follicular atresia). The genitalia are hypotrophic, and the immature uterus has a thin mucosa, with poorly developed glands. The mammary glands have rudimentary ducts, with no secretory acini.

C. FROM PUBERTY TO MENOPAUSE

Puberty is characterized by the onset of cyclic hormonal activity. The *releasing hormones* of the hypothalamus stimulate the hypophysis to secrete FSH and LH. FSH and LH determine ovarian modifications, which in turn are responsible for changes in the genital ducts. The uterus, vagina, vulva, and breasts remain in an immature stage until they develop under the influence of estrogens originating in the ovary. Estrogen is responsible for the appearance of pubic and axillary hair.

I. Ovaries

At puberty, under the stimulus of FSH and LH, the first menstrual cycle occurs. These cycles repeat about every 28 days until menopause. The first few cycles, as well as the last few, are frequently anovulatory.

Preovulation Phase

During the first 14 days of the menstrual cycle, several follicles grow and differentiate. Only one reaches maturation, under the stimulation of

FSH. Differentiation occurs in primitive oocytes arrested in the prophase stage of the first meiotic division.

a. Oocytes. *The oocyte* hypertrophies as the cytoplasm increases in volume and fills with lipid droplets. A clear layer, the zona pellucida, appears at the periphery of the ovum. At the end of its development, the oocyte has an approximate diameter of 150 μm. The first meiotic division, begun years earlier, ends shortly before ovulation and gives rise to two cells—the secondary oocyte and the first polar body.

b. The Peripheral Cells. These are of two types:

Follicular cells, satellites of the oocyte, are devoid of vascularization and hormonal activity during the first part of the ovarian cycle.

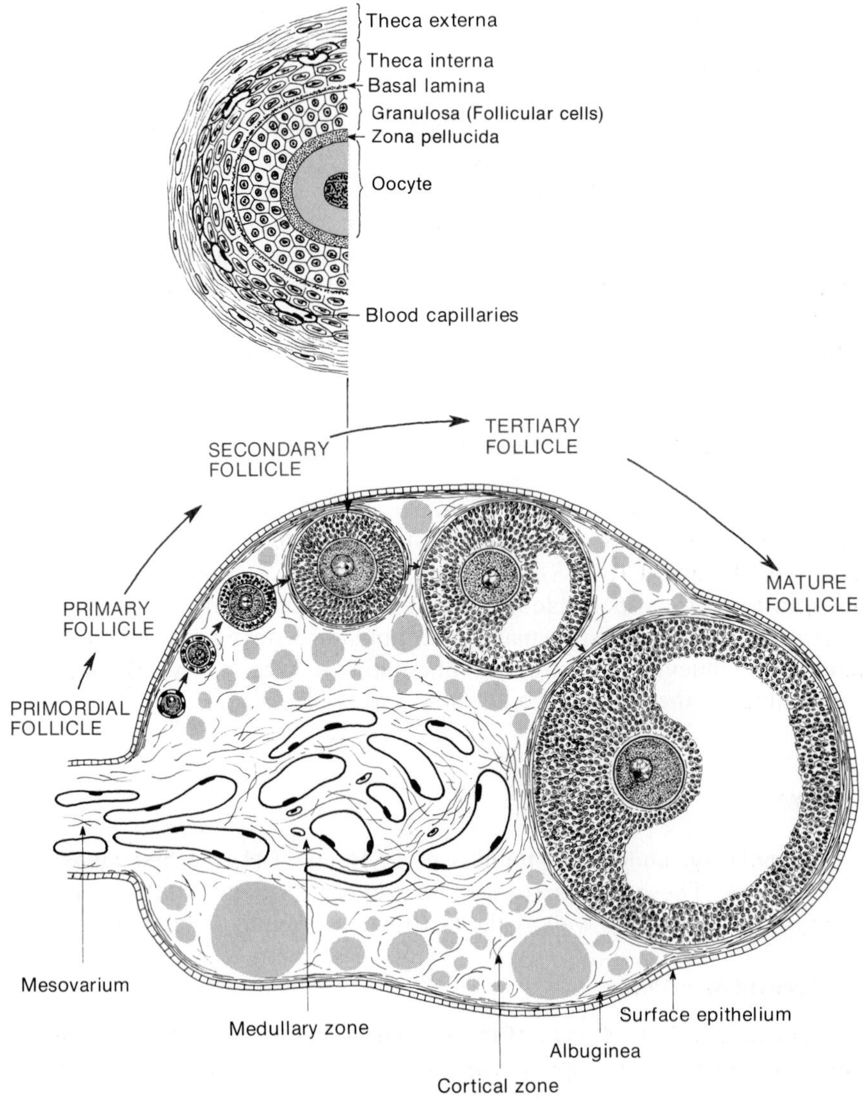

Figure 97. Schematic structure of the ovary (at the end of the preovulatory phase).

During maturation of the follicle, the granulosa cells multiply and form many layers around the oocyte. Cavities between cells fill with a fluid and merge to form a single central cavity. The oocyte, surrounded by a single cellular layer (future corona radiata), attaches itself at the periphery of the follicle.

The cells of the ovarian stroma (mesenchymal in origin) multiply at the periphery of the granulosa, from which they are separated by a thick basal lamina, to form the *theca interna.* These well-vascularized epithelium-like cells secrete the estrogens responsible for uterine and vaginal modifications during this first half of the cycle. The *theca externa,* also well vascularized, is essentially connective tissue with no hormonal activity.

Thus, in the course of growth and maturation (during which a primordial follicle, with an original diameter of 25 μm, develops to the mature stage, with a diameter of 10 to 55 mm), the oocyte and the peripheral cells undergo important modifications. However, only the theca interna is functional and only one type of hormone (estrogens) is secreted.

Ovulation

On the fourteenth day of the cycle, the sudden increase in LH secretion, acting upon a mature follicle, liberates the oocyte with its zona pellucida and corona radiata. At that time, it is a haploid cell (secondary oocyte) whose first meiotic division terminated prior to ovulation. The mature follicle, bulging at the thinned, avascular surface, ruptures, and the oocyte is flushed out by follicular fluid. The exact mechanism of follicular rupture is unknown (vascular phenomenon? enzymatic lysis?). The walls of the ruptured follicle in the ovary collapse around a residual serofibrinous exudate, forming a temporary endocrine gland, the corpus luteum.

Postovulatory Phase

The secondary oocyte, which was discharged from the ovary, is captured by the fimbriae of the oviduct. If fertilization fails to occur, the oocyte degenerates rapidly, and the corpus luteum, responsible for modification of the genital tract, is established. The capillaries of the theca interna extend beyond the basal lamina which separates them from the granulosa. The granulosa cells undergo differentiation and present the typical aspect of steroid secreting cells. Two hormones then appear: (1) *Progesterone,* secreted by the large lutein cells of the granulosa cells, and (2) *estrogens,* secreted by cells of the theca interna which have become small lutein cells. With no barrier between granulosa and theca interna cells, they become highly vascularized, forming the corpus luteum. The periodically formed corpus luteum has a precise life span. Fourteen days after ovulation, it suddenly stops secretion, and this hormonal deprivation sets off the beginning of menstruation. All that remains in the ovary to demarcate the site of a corpus luteum is a fibrous scar, the corpus albicans.

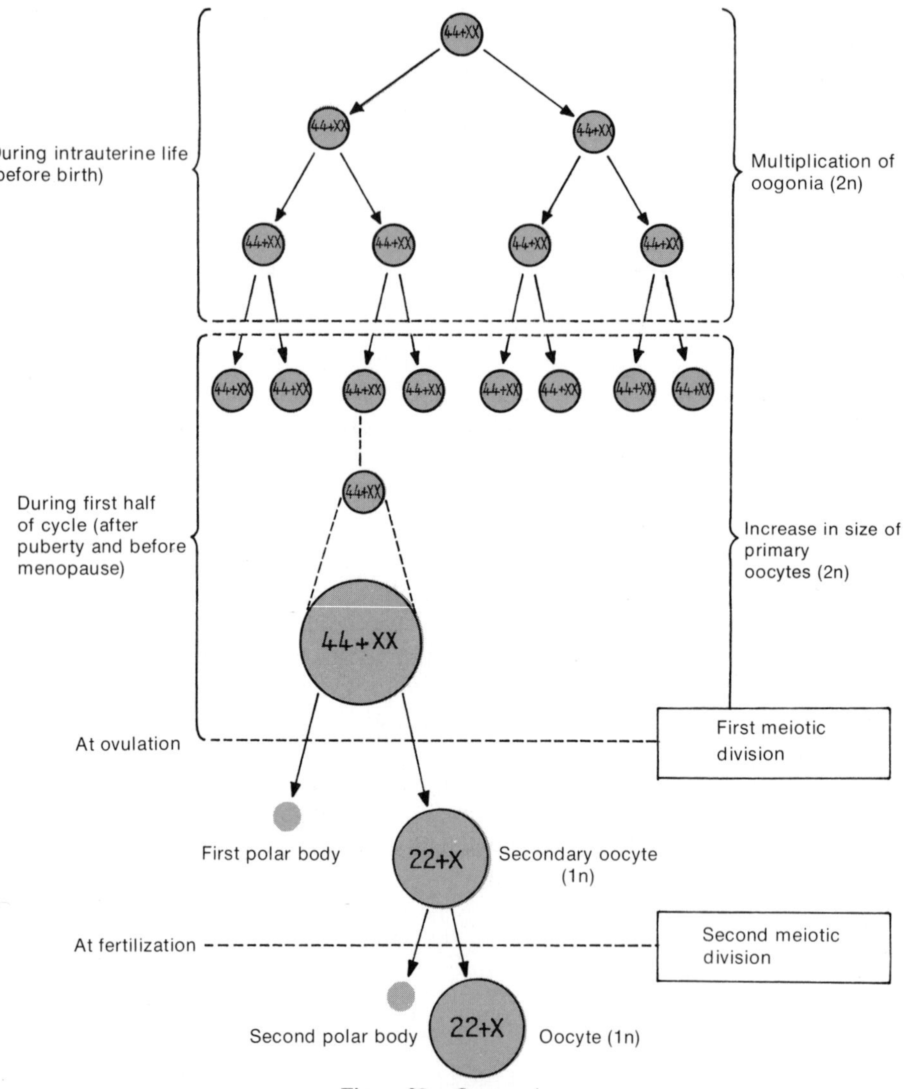

Figure 98. Oogenesis.

II. The Uterus and Menstruation

Mucosa of the Uterine Body (Endometrium)

The modifications in the uterine mucosa (menstrual cycle) are due to the isolated action of estrogens, and followed by the joint action of estrogens and progesterone. There are three successive phases:

a. Proliferative Phase. The uterine mucosa, shed by hemorrhagic necrosis during menstruation, regenerates from the intact deep layer. From the fourth to fourteenth days of the cycle, there are numerous mitoses in the cells of the glands and of the lamina propria. The glands grow, but retain their straight tubular shape, and vessels develop. Glycogen droplets appear in the basal cytoplasm of glandular cells. This growth phase is associated with estrogen secretion by the ovary.

b. Secretory Phase. At ovulation, progesterone begins to work along with estrogens. Mitoses progressively diminish in the lamina propria and in the glands. Glycogen accumulates at the apical pole of the glandular cells. These tubular convoluted glands confer on the endometrium the classic structure described as "uterine lace." Vessel development is considerable and branches of coiled arterioles reach the most superficial part of the mucosa. The lamina propria is edematous, and some cells become decidual.

c. Menstrual Phase. Shortly before menstruation, rhythmic contractions of the superficial arterioles set in. These contractions become increasingly lengthy. Closing of arteriovenous shunts is said to be responsible for

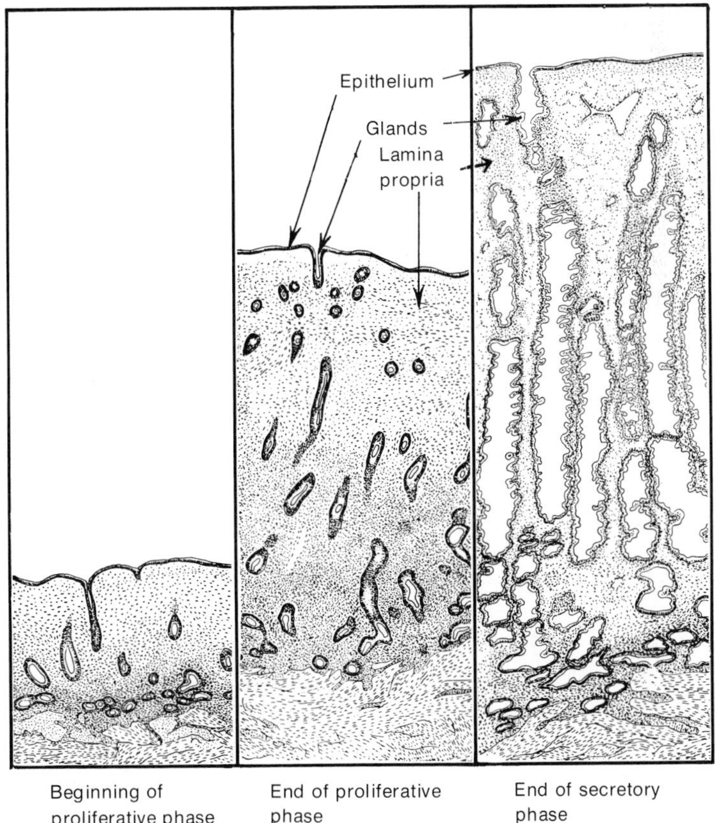

Figure 99. The uterine mucosa during the menstrual cycle (×30). (Modified after O. Bucher, 1972.)

the localized ischemic necroses which take place successively from one zone to another. These necroses provoke a hemorrhage, termed menstruation (blood mixed with endometrial debris), which lasts several days. These phenomena are due to sudden hormonal deprivation, which can be reproduced artificially.

Mucosa of the Uterine Cervix

Secretory cells of the epithelium of the inner cervix and endocervical glands are subject to estrogen influence from the very start of the cycle. They secrete abundant mucous material during the days preceding ovulation. The quality of this mucus affects the motility of the spermatozoa, which is indispensable for their ascension towards the uterine cavity.

Vaginal Epithelium

Histological modifications of vaginal epithelium are linked to the ovarian secretions (estrogen and progesterone). The unique desquamation of this epithelium forms the basis of the cytological modifications seen in "vaginal smears." The percentage of eosinophilic cells (eosinophilic index) and the percentage of dense pyknotic nuclei (pyknotic index) having a diameter of 6 μm or less give some indication of the degree of estrogenic effect. Vaginal cytology tests have lost much of their value with increased use of contraceptive pills; the main purpose of vaginal or cervical smears (Pap test) is the early detection of uterine cancer.

The Breasts

Estrogenic secretion, during the first cycles of puberty, stimulates proliferation of the mammary ducts, development of interlobar and interlobular connective tissue, and increase in adipose tissue. Except during pregnancy and breast feeding, the mammary glands are in a resting state. Only a few acini develop during the second part of the menstrual cycle, under the influence of progesterone.

D. DURING PREGNANCY

I. Ovaries

If the ovum is fertilized, it becomes a zygote, undergoes the second meiotic (equational) division, sheds it second polar body, and starts the first segmentational divisions.

The corpus luteum becomes the corpus luteum of pregnancy, elaborating estrogens and progesterone through the first months of pregnancy. Maturation of ovarian follicles ceases in both ovaries, and is resumed only when secretion of FSH is renewed some time after parturition.

II. Structures Affected by Ovarian Hormones

Corpus Uteri

a. The Endometrium. The endometrium undergoes important modifications following implantation of the ovum. Cells of the lamina propria are transformed into the decidua parietalis. After delivery, the endometrium is restored in the same way as after the menstrual phase.

b. The Myometrium. The myometrium, under the influence of estrogen, undergoes considerable hypertrophy, linked to the increase in number and volume of the smooth muscle cells.

Cervix Uteri

Cervical secretions cease at ovulation, and the cervical canal is obstructed by a "mucous plug."

Vaginal Epithelium

The modifications of the vaginal epithelium are linked to an abundant progesterone secretion. Vaginal smears show increasingly atrophic cells during pregnancy. "Navicular" or "pregnancy" cells appear.

Breasts

During the first half of pregnancy, under the influence of progesterone, a great number of glandular acini develop from terminal ramifications of the duct system. In the first months of gestation, prolactin stimulates glandular acini to secrete a product rich in proteins and poor in lipids (colostrum). In the days following delivery, milk secretion begins owing to the increase of prolactin secretion. It is maintained because of a neurohormonal reflex stimulated by infant suckling. During the entire suckling period, the mammary gland is in a state of "lactation." The epithelium of the acini presents distinct signs of secretory activity: tall columnar cells with an accumulation of lipid droplets and secretory granules. The lumina of the acini and ducts are filled with milk, which distends them. Under the electron microscope, the acinar cells display protein granules (which originate in the granular endoplasmic reticulum, are packaged by the Golgi complex, and are discharged by exocytosis) and lipid droplets, packaged in a cytoplasmic membrane (apocrine secretion). Ejection of milk during suckling is initiated by a neurohormonal reflex set off by mechanical stimulation of the nipple. This starts contraction of the myoepithelial cells surrounding the acini, and accumulated milk in the acini is ejected into lactiferous sinuses, from where it is released at the nipple. After lactation, the mammary gland progressively resumes its resting condition, without, however, recovering its exact initial state; many of the acini formed during pregnancy do not disappear completely.

E. AFTER MENOPAUSE

Of the 400,000 primordial ova present at birth, 99.9 per cent progress to one or another of the stages of maturation and degenerate, and only about 0.1 per cent (about 400) are released at ovulation. After menopause, no follicles remain. Only a few *corpora albicantia* may persist in the fibrous tissue.

After menopause, the endometrium undergoes progressive atrophy; the lumina of the glands become occluded and form cysts. The vaginal epithelium also undergoes atrophy and progressive involution. The remaining acini of the mammary glands have a tendency to revert to their prepubertal state.

19

Endocrine Glands

A. HYPOPHYSIS

I. Parts of the Hypophysis

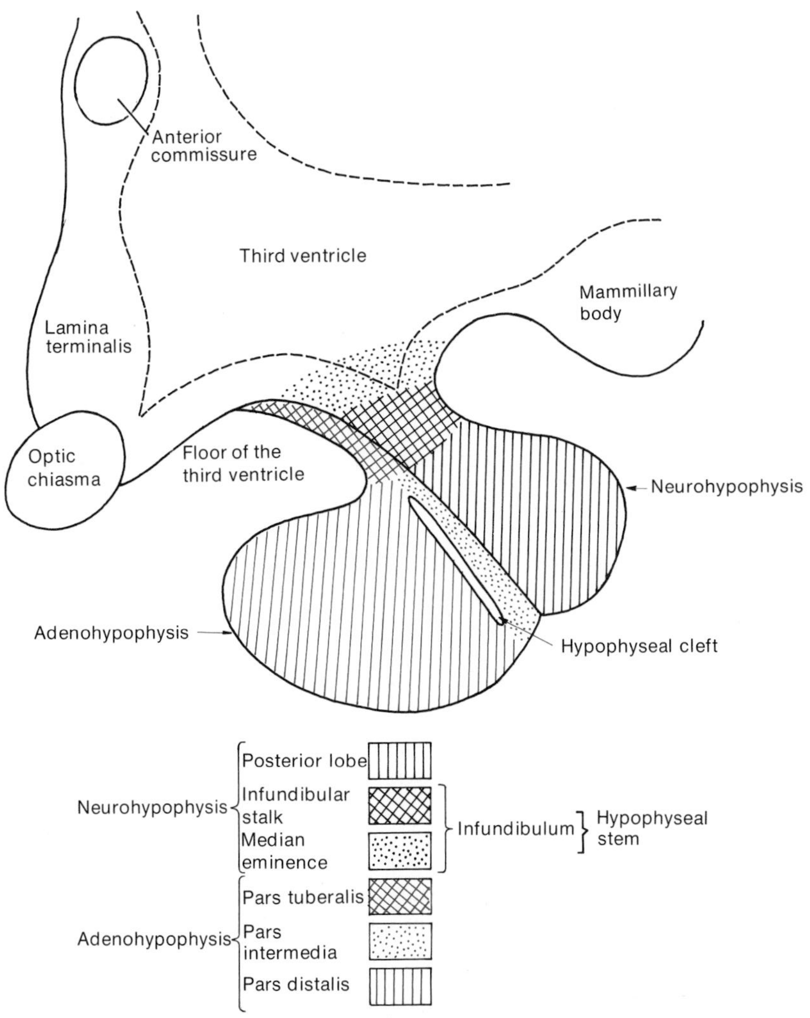

Figure 100. Parts of the hypophysis.

II. Adenohypophysis

Anterior Lobe

The anterior lobe, comprising the major portion of the adenohypophysis and enclosed in a delicate connective tissue capsule, is made of endocrine glandular cells in a rich network of fenestrated blood capillaries.

a. Cells of Anterior Lobe. *There are seven cell types corresponding to the seven adenohypophyseal hormones: TSH cells, FSH cells, LH cells, MSH cells, STH cells, ACTH cells, and prolactin cells.* These different cell types can be distinguished with the light microscope only after special stains. Usual stains (hematoxylin and eosin) distinguish only three cell types (acidophils, basophils, and chromophobes) and provide little histophysiological correlation. With the electron microscope, all adenohypophyseal cells show organelles involved in synthesis and secretion of polypeptides (ACTH and MSH), pure proteins (STH and prolactin), and glycoproteins (TSH, FSH, LH). The distribution of these organelles, plus the size, number, and character of the secretory granules, provides morphological distinction of the various cell types.

The proportions of these seven cell types vary according to physiological conditions (such as pregnancy, parturition, menopause, and so forth). There is no clear systemization for their distribution in humans.

b. Secretions of Anterior Lobe. The secretory activity of the adenohypophyseal cells is regulated by neurohormones (*releasing* or *inhibitory factors* secreted by neurons in the lateral wall of the hypothalamus). The releasing and inhibitory factors are polypeptides of low molecular weight. Some factors activate, others inhibit adenohypophyseal secretion. Eight are known at the present time. These hypothalamic hormones reach adenohypophyseal cells via the hypophyseal portal system. This system consists of: (1) *afferent arteries,* which are the superior hypophyseal arteries from the internal carotids, narrowing into (2) *a first capillary network,* located in the median eminence, into which the axons of the hypothalamic neurons secrete their neurohormones; this capillary network is drained by (3) *hypophyseal portal veins,* which run transversely to the pituitary stalk, giving rise to (4) *a second capillary network,* located within the adenohypophysis; hypothalamic hormones reach the adenohypophyseal glandular cells to stimulate or inhibit them, and the adenohypophyseal hormones are then secreted into the second capillary network and reach (5) *efferent veins,* consisting of hypophyseal veins that terminate in the internal jugular vein.

Intermediate Lobe

The intermediate lobe is extremely small and its role in humans is unknown. Melanocyte stimulating hormone (MSH) is probably secreted by cells of the intermediate lobe.

TABLE 30. Hypophysiotropic Hypothalamic Neurohormones

Adenohypophyseal Hormones		GH or STH	TSH	ACTH	MSH	LH/ICSH and FSH	Prolactin
Hypophysiotropic Hypothalamic Neurohormones	Releasing Factors (RF)	GH-RF	TSH-RF	ACTH-RF	MSH-RF	LH/ICSH- and FSH-RF	
	Inhibiting Factors (IF)	GH-IF			MSH-IF		PIF

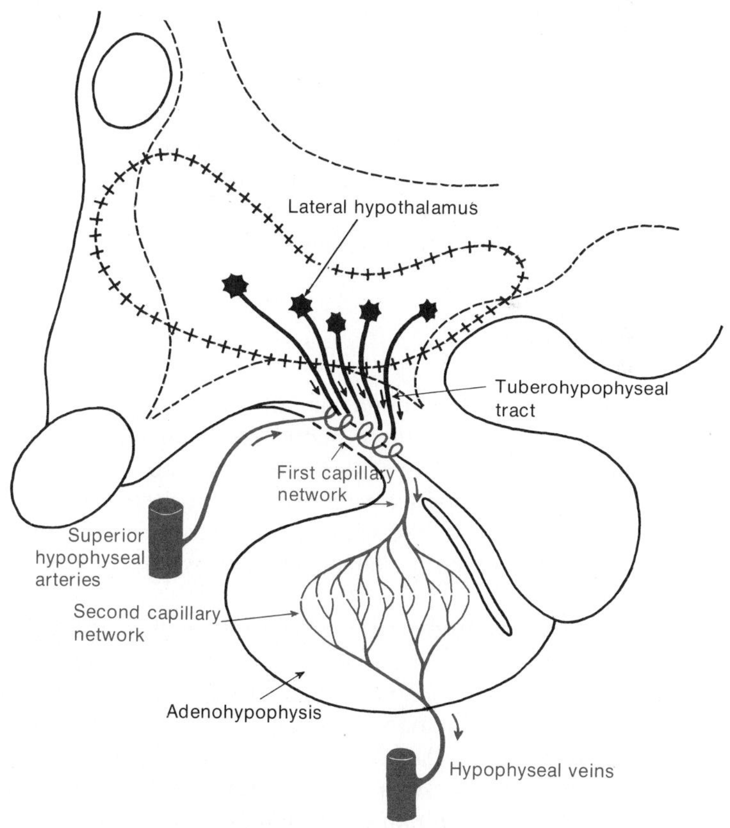

Figure 101. Adenohypophysis.

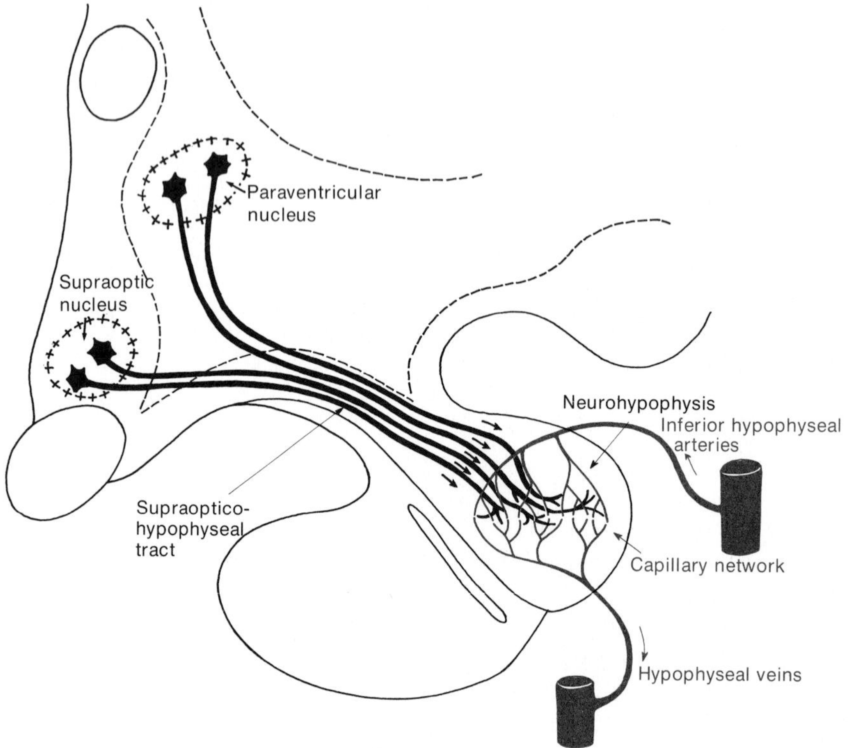

Figure 102. Neurohypophysis.

III. Neurohypophysis

The posterior lobe (neurohypophysis) of the hypophysis does not secrete neurohormones. Instead, these peptide hormones are synthesized by certain hypothalamic neurons whose axons reach the neurohypophysis and release their secretory product into its capillary network. Thus, antidiuretic hormone (ADH) is synthesized by the neurons of the supraoptic nuclei and possibly the paraventricular nuclei, and oxytocin by neurons of the paraventricular nuclei.

The structure of the neurohypophysis consists mainly of blood capillaries and axons of neurons from supraoptic and paraventricular nuclei. Glial cells (or pituicytes), similar to astrocytes of the central nervous system, are located between the axons. Using special stains, neurosecretory granules may be seen within the axons. Often they form spherical aggregates, the Herring bodies. With the electron microscope, secretory granules appear like vesicles with an electron-dense core.

Unlike the portal system of the adenohypophysis, the neurohypophysis possesses only a regular capillary network rising from the inferior hypophyseal arteries. The capillary network is drained by hypophyseal veins, which flow into the internal jugular vein.

B. THYROID

The thyroid is a lobulated endocrine gland made up of thyroid follicles located in a vascular connective tissue stroma rich in fenestrated blood capillaries. Thyroid follicles are spherical formations consisting of: (1) a wall of simple epithelium resting on a basal lamina and consisting of two cell types—follicular cells and C (thyrocalcitonin) cells; and (2) an amorphous content (colloid) which is pasty and yellowish when fresh.

I. Follicular Cells

The follicular cells (or thyrocytes) secrete the thyroid hormones triiodothyronine and tetraiodothyronine or thyroxin.

The basal poles of follicular cells rest on the basal lamina of the follicle, and the apical poles project microvilli into the colloid. The lateral surfaces join adjacent follicular cells via junctional complexes. These cells possess a basal or central nucleus, mitochondria, granular endoplasmic reticulum, ribosomes, a supranuclear Golgi complex, numerous lysosomes, phagosomes ("colloid droplets"), and phagolysosomes. Follicular cells vary according to their degree of activity. In *hyperactivity,* their volume increases, they become tall columnar, and their organelles undergo consider-

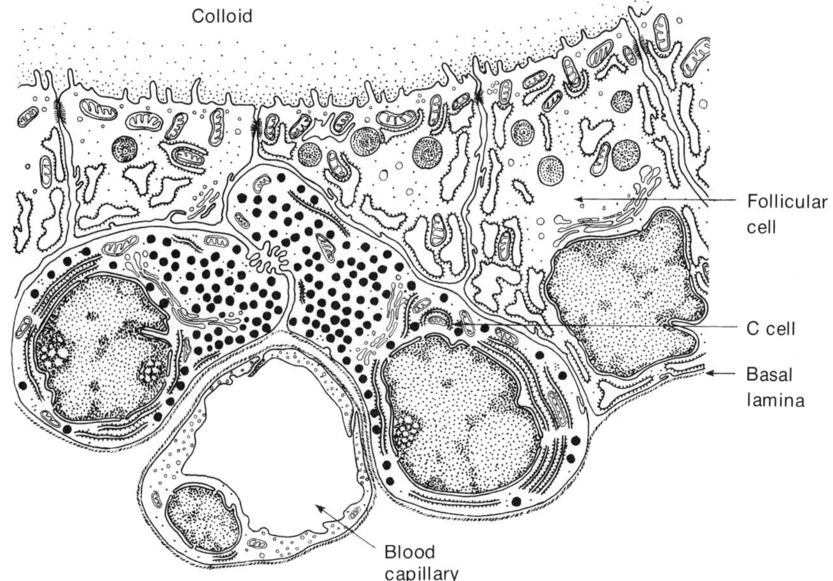

Figure 103. Electron microscopic diagram of C cells of the thyroid. (After A. G. E. Pearse and U. Welsch, 1968.)

able development. At the same time, the volume and stainability of colloid diminishes or it may even disappear completely. In *hypoactivity,* these phenomena are reversed: the thyrocytes become smaller and cuboidal or even flattened, organelles diminish, and the colloid increases in volume and becomes very acidophilic.

Follicular cells capture the blood iodides (actively, necessitating a strong energy expenditure) and release them into the colloid, where they are concentrated and oxidized.

In addition, the follicular cell synthesizes the glycoprotein thyroglobulin. The protein fraction is synthesized by ribosomes in the granular endoplasmic reticulum from amino acids (tyrosine) of the blood. It then passes into the Golgi complex where the carbohydrate fraction is synthesized and added to it. The Golgi vesicles migrate to the apical surface of the cell and release the thyroglobulin via exocytosis into the follicular lumen, where it contributes to colloid formation.

Iodine in the colloid is then incorporated in the thyroglobulin as monoiodotyrosines (MIT) *and diiodotyrosines* (DIT), which later condense to triiodothyronine and tetraiodothyronine.

The colloid (iodinated thyroglobulin) is later phagocytized by the follicular cells, to form intracytoplasmic colloid droplets (phagosomes). Lysosomes gravitate to the colloid droplets and form phagolysosomes. Iodinated thyroglobulin is degraded by acid hydrolysis and liberates triiodo- and tetraiodothyronine, as well as residual iodotyrosines (MIT and DIT). Triiodo- and tetraiodothyronines, which were freed inside the follicular cell, are released into the blood capillaries surrounding the follicles. The residual iodotyrosines are deiodinated in situ in the follicular cell, and yield (1) tyrosine, which returns to the blood capillaries and contributes to the pool of circulating amino acids, and (2) mineral iodine, which enters the iodine cycle, either being reutilized immediately or returning to the blood circulation.

II. C Cells

Less numerous than the thyrocytes, the C cells are located against the basal lamina of the follicles but are never in contact with colloid. Via electron microscopy they are characterized mainly by the presence of numerous cytoplasmic electron-dense membrane-bound granules. These calcitonin secreting granules (polypeptide hormones) are later freed by exocytosis and are taken up by adjacent blood capillaries.

C. PARATHYROID GLANDS

The endocrine glandular cells of the parathyroid are grouped in cords or clumps around connective tissue rich in adipose cells and fenestrated blood capillaries. They synthesize and secrete into the blood (following the general patterns of protein secretion) the parathyroid hormone or parathormone, (which is of polypeptide nature). The rate of secretion is in direct proportion to the level of ionized calcium in the blood.

Large oxyphilic cells, rich in mitochondria, are found in varying numbers in the parathyroid parenchyma. These cells increase in number with advancing age; however, their role is unknown.

D. SUPRARENAL GLANDS

I. The Adrenal Cortex

The constituting elements of the adrenal cortex (glandular cells, fenestrated capillaries, and connective tissue network) are arranged in three zones. Beginning with the outermost these are: (1) *zona glomerulosa,* in which the cells are arranged in more or less rounded clusters; (2) *zona fasciculata,* in which the cells are arranged in long cords perpendicular to the surface; and (3) *zona reticularis,* in which the cells form a network of anastomosing cords.

Glandular cells secrete cortical steroid hormones into the blood. Despite minor differences, cells of the cortical zones present morphological characteristics like those of steroid secreting cells: smooth endoplasmic reticulum, mitochondria with tubular cristae, liposomes, and lipofuscin pigment.

Localization of enzymes responsible for biosynthesis of these hormones is well known. Mitochondria contain enzymes that split off the lateral chain of cholesterol (leading to the Δ5-pregnenolone), as well as 11B-hydroxylase and 18-aldolase, which permit the final stages in synthesis of corticosterone and aldosterone. The smooth endoplasmic reticulum contains enzymes responsible for the biosynthesis of cholesterol from acetate, as well as numerous enzymes controlling synthesis of progesterone, androgens, and intermediate products leading to cortisol.

Summary

Aldosterone is secreted by cells of the zona glomerulosa which are the only cells containing 18-aldolase (an enzyme which facilitates passage of corticosterone to aldosterone). Secretion of aldosterone is controlled by *renin.*

Glucocorticoids (cortisol and cortisone) *as well as suprarenal androgens* (mainly dehydroepiandrosterone) are secreted by cells of the zona fasciculata and zona reticularis, but it is not possible to state with certainty whether the cells of these two zones are specialized for the synthesis of these two groups of hormones. Secretion of glucocorticoids is regulated by *ACTH,* and secretion of suprarenal androgens is controlled by *ACTH* and *LH.*

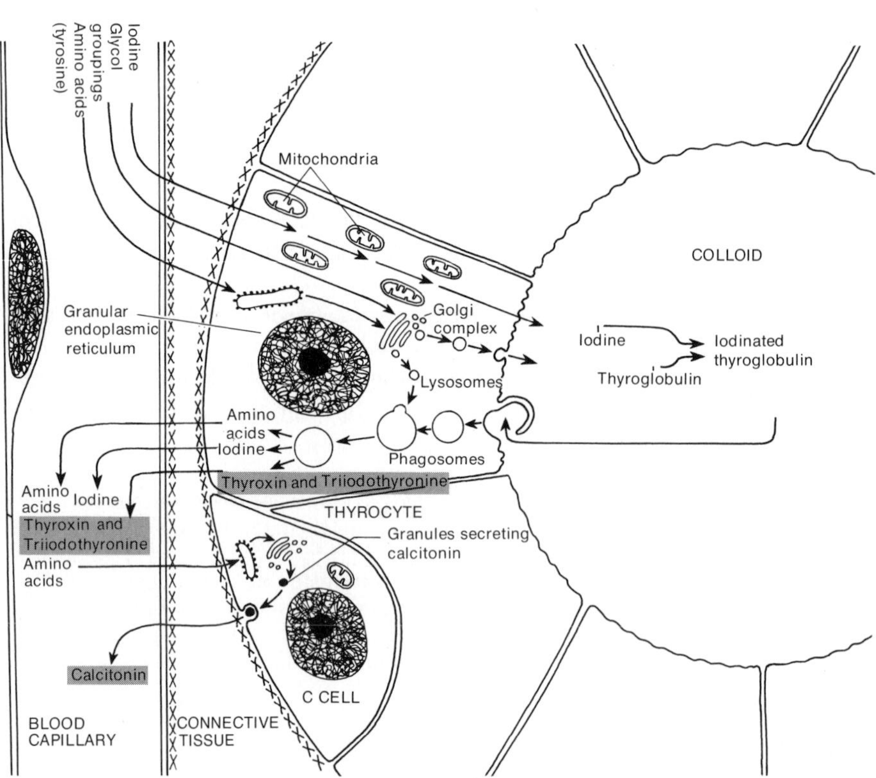

Figure 104. Diagram of an elaboration of thyroid hormones (triiodo- and tetraiiodothyronine) and of calcitonin.

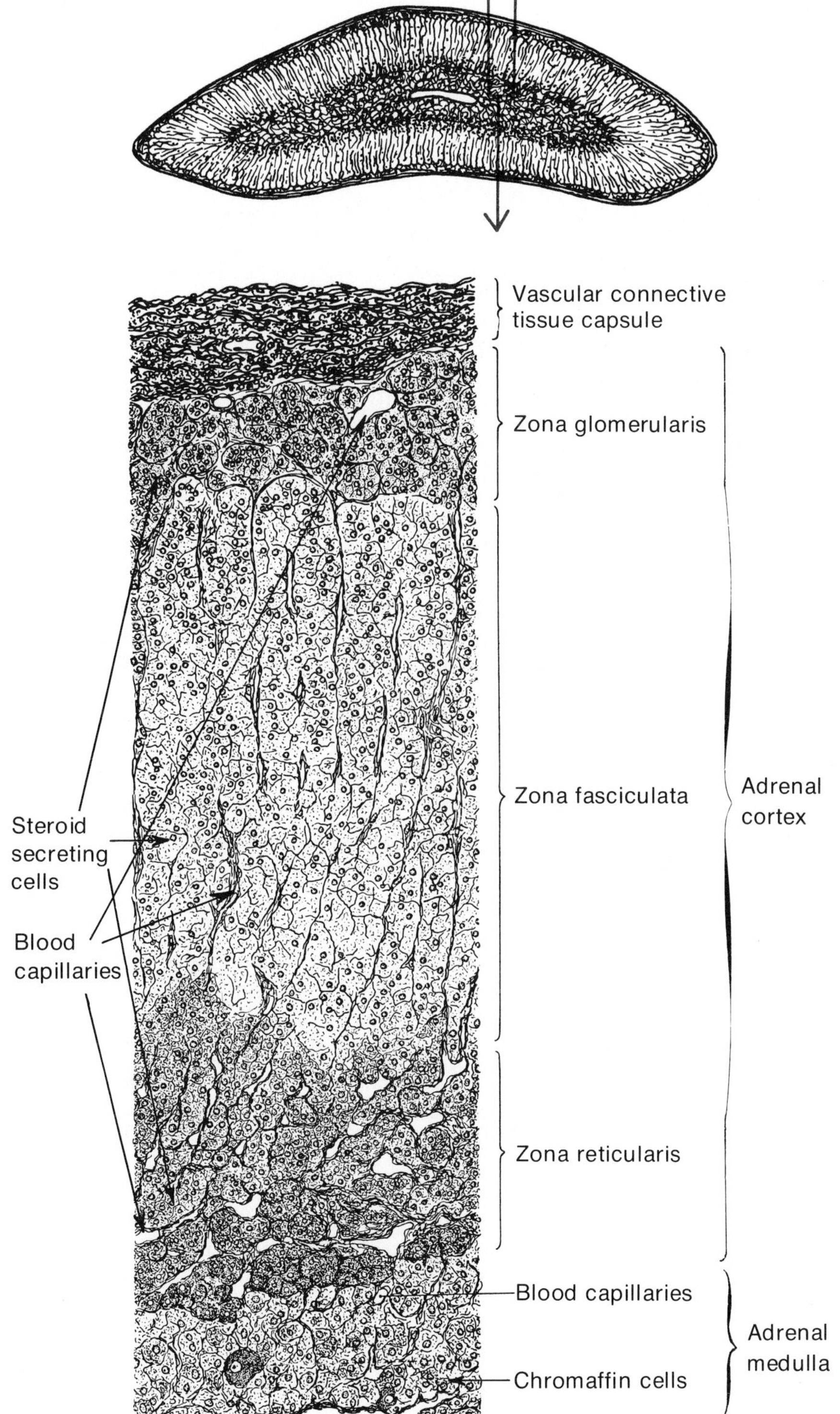

Figure 105. Different zones of the suprarenal gland. (After O. Bucher, 1973.)

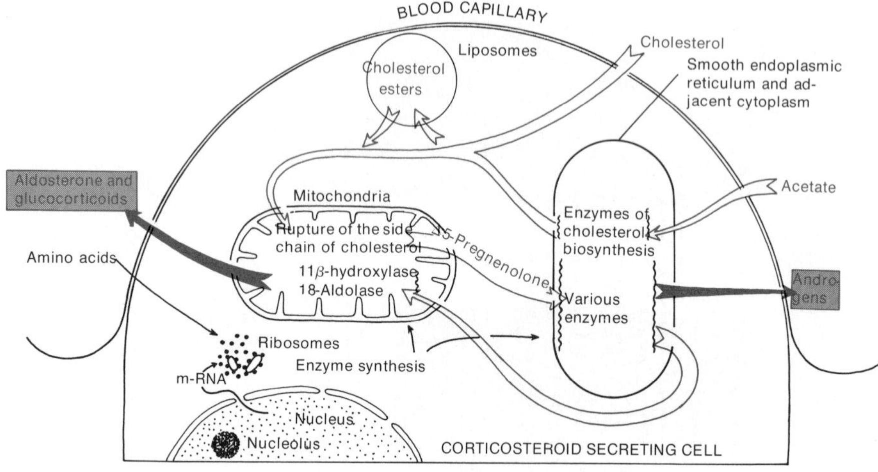

Figure 106. Synthesis of suprarenal cortical hormones.

II. Adrenal Medulla

The adrenal medulla, located in the center of the adrenal cortex, is made of cords of large polyhedral glandular cells, between which are fenestrated blood capillaries surrounded by a thin connective tissue network.

Cells of the Medulla

The glandular cells of the adrenal medulla are characterized by the presence in their cytoplasm of numerous small, membrane-bound electron-dense granules, which are the granules secreting catecholamines.* In some cells these granules contain norepinephrine, but most of the cells secrete epinephrine. Histochemical and ultrastructural criteria allow one to distinguish epinephrine cells from norepinephrine cells. In both types the procedures of synthesis, storage, and excretion are analogous. Three of the four synthesized enzymes are in the cytoplasm; only dopamine-β-hydroxylase, which transforms dopamine into norepinephrine, is located at the level of the secretory granules. These have enzymatic sites and a storage compartment for norepinephrine or epinephrine (depending on the type of cell). Secretory granules are excreted by exocytosis into the blood capillaries of the adrenal medulla.

Secretions

The volume of secretion and excretion depends on nervous stimuli from the cholinergic axons of sympathetic protoneurons that form a synaptic

*The secretory granules, which are barely visible with the light microscope with usual stains, appear larger and brown in color when fixed with various oxidizing agents, particularly chromium salts (from which they receive the name *chromaffin* or *pheochrome cells*).

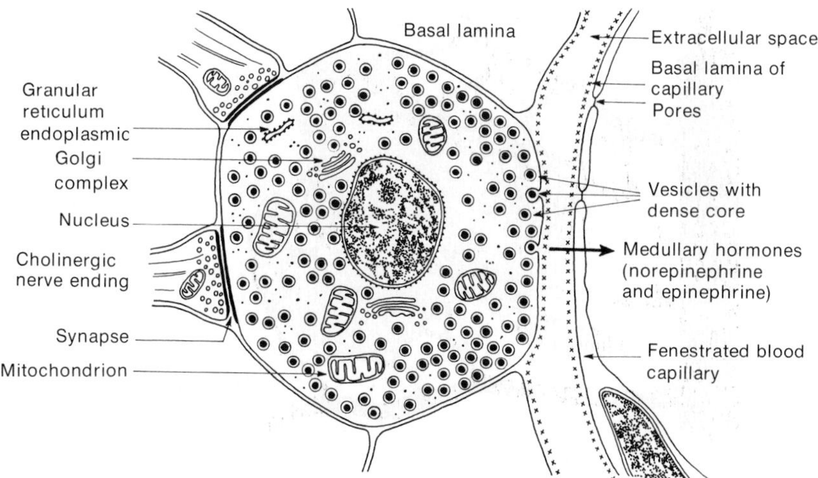

Figure 107. Schematic ultrastructural representation of a chromaffin cell of the adrenal medulla.

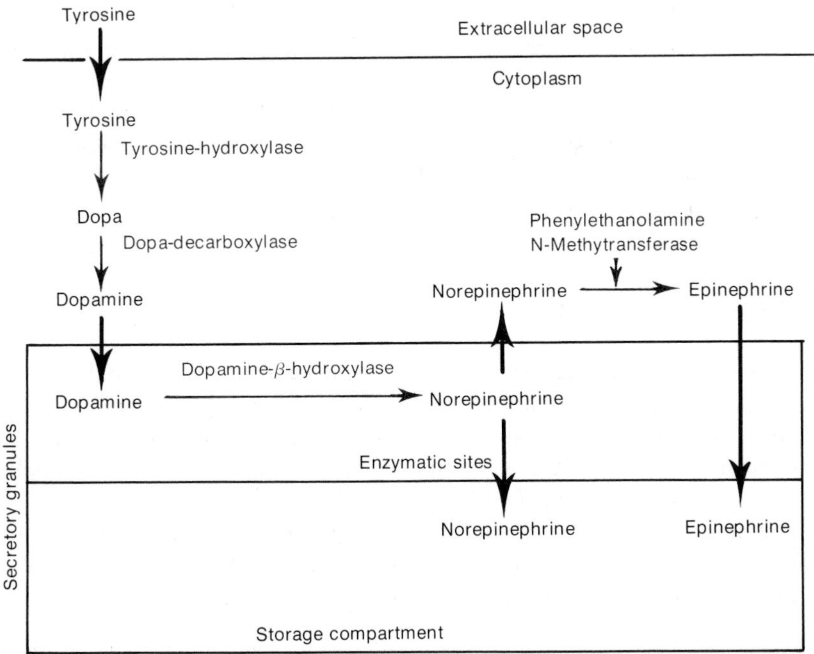

Figure 108. Mechanism of synthesis of catecholamines in chromaffin cells of the adrenal medulla. (After Stjärne, 1972.)

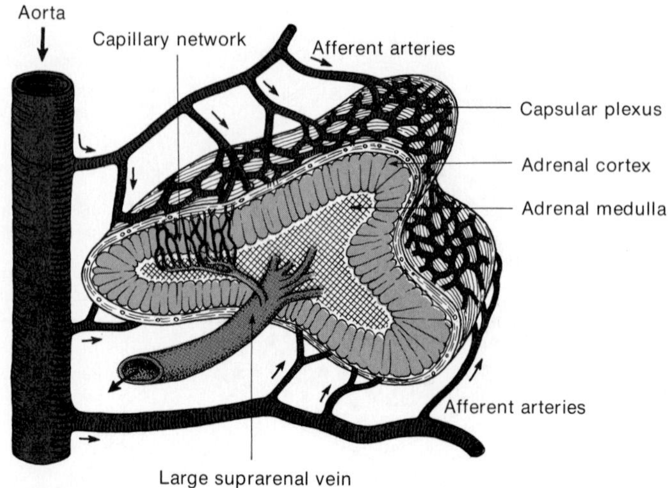

Figure 109. Vascularization of the adrenal. (After H. Elias and J. E. Pauly, 1966.)

junction on the membrane of the glandular cells. The glucocorticoids also participate in this control, since they are essential for the activity of the phenylethanolamine-N-methyltransferase, which permits the methylation of norepinephrine into epinephrine. The importance of this hormonal control is demonstrated by the dual blood supply to the adrenal medulla. It is supplied by blood coming for the most part from the capillary network which traversed the adrenal cortex, which, therefore, contains adrenocortical hormones (Fig. 109), and a direct arterial supply.

E. PINEAL (EPIPHYSIS)

At the superior posterior part of the third ventricle is the epiphysis (or pineal gland) made of pinealocytes, glial cells of astrocyte type, and blood capillaries surrounded by a perivascular space containing some collagenous fibers. Numerous sympathetic axons, from the superior cervical ganglia, form synaptic junctions on the glandular cells.

Pinealocytes synthesize and secrete the hormone melatonin into the blood. This product is visible electron microscopically as spherical secretory granules with an electron-dense core.

Synthesis of melatonin is initiated by serotonin (which is synthesized by the pinealocytes from tryptophan drawn from the blood), and catalyzed by a specific enzyme, 5-HIOMT (5-hydroxyindole-O-methyltransferase). Synthesis of melatonin is under photic control—darkness increases it, light diminishes it. It has been found that light signals are transmitted by axons of the superior cervical sympathetic

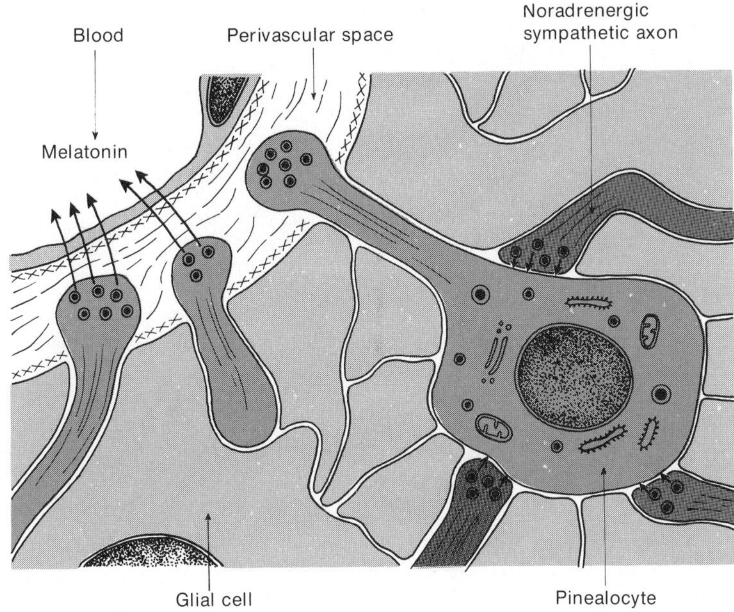

Figure 110. Schematic representation of the pineal gland as seen with the electron microscope.

ganglia. Norepinephrine freed by their endings seems to act, under the influence of cyclic AMP, upon the degree of activity of the 5-HIOMT of the pinealocytes and, therefore, upon the rate of melatonin synthesis.

It is known that melatonin has a strong effect on the retraction of cutaneous melanophores of amphibians, and it also has the capacity to restrict gonadal function. Its exact physiological role in humans is unknown.

F. PANCREATIC ISLETS OF LANGERHANS

The islets of Langerhans are small cellular masses supplied by an abundant network of fenestrated blood capillaries.

In routine histological specimens, they appear as small, rounded, lightly staining masses, arranged without order and in variable numbers inside the pancreatic lobules.

The endocrine glandular cells, which make up these masses, are of three types (B, A_2, A_1) and are distinguishable only after special staining (fuchsin–paraldehyde; hematoxylin–chrome–phloxine; metachromatic reactions; argentaffin reactions). They are easily recognizable electron microscopically by the size and density of their secretory granules.

Considerable histochemical, immunological (fluorescent antibodies), physiological, pharmacological, and pathological evidence has led to the conclusion that *B cells secrete insulin; A_2 cells secrete glucagon; and A_1 cells secrete gastrin.* Secretory mechanisms for these three cell types are similar to the general mechanisms involved in synthesis and secretion of other protein and polypeptide hormones.

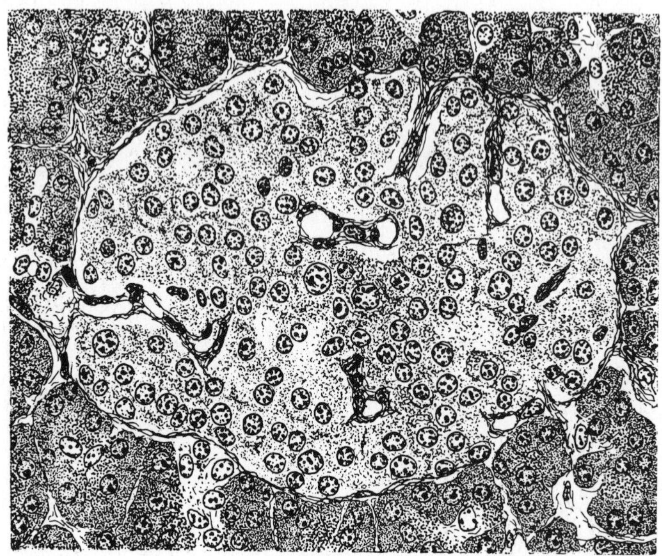

Figure 111. Pancreatic islets of Langerhans, surrounded by exocrine acini (×500). (After O. Bucher, 1973.)

Sympathetic and parasympathetic innervation of the islets of Langerhans is well developed. Neuronal cell bodies are sometimes visible.

Like exocrine acini, the islets of Langerhans rise from the proliferation of cells in the extremities of primitive entodermal pancreatic diverticula. Under certain physiological or experimental conditions, new islets may arise from the cells of the acini or of the excretory ducts (insular neogenesis). Regression is also possible (insular retrogenesis).

20

Skin and Sense Organs

I. THE SKIN

A. THE LAYERS OF SKIN

The skin is made up of three layers: epidermis, dermis, and hypodermis.

I. EPIDERMIS

The outermost layer, the epidermis, is a stratified squamous epithelium composed of three different cell lineages: keratinocytes, melanocytes, and stellate epidermal cells (Langerhans cells). It contains no blood or lymph vessels, but has numerous sensitive nerve endings (free nerve endings and Merkel's corpuscles).

Keratinocytes

The keratinocytes undergo a continuous morphological evolution leading to their keratinization. These changes progress from the basal layers to the surface. In a section of epidermis, four layers can be distinguished from the basal lamina outward. The first or deepest layer (*stratum basale* or germinative layer) is responsible for the continual renewal of the epidermis by mitoses. These cells, which are cuboidal or columnar, contain numerous phagocytized melanin granules, conferring on the epidermis a protective role against light and contributing to the keratinocyte's regulation of cutaneous pigmentation.

In the overlying layers, important progressive modifications of the cells take place, leading to complete keratinization of the superficial layers and providing a protective barrier (mechanical and chemical) for the epidermis.

In the *stratum spinosum* (second layer) the cells begin to flatten, but nuclear and cytoplasmic organelles remain intact. Tonofilaments are grouped in dense fascicles, and desmosomes are prominent. The cells of the *stratum granulosum* (third layer) are flattened, and their nuclei begin to degenerate. Most importantly, numerous granules of keratohyalin can be found within the meshwork of tonofilaments. Finally, in the *stratum corneum* (outermost layer) the cells are completely flattened, nuclear and cytoplasmic organelles have completely disappeared, and the cytoplasm is filled with bundles of keratin fibers (formed from the tonofilaments and keratohyalin granules). The plasma membranes have become very dense and flattened, and desmosomes undergo a profound modification. At the surface of the stratum corneum, fully keratinized dead cells become detached from the epidermis and are shed (desquamation).

Frequently there is a clear layer, the *stratum lucidum,* interposed between the granulosum and corneum. It is most prominent in thick skin. Eleidin granules are found in these flattened cells.

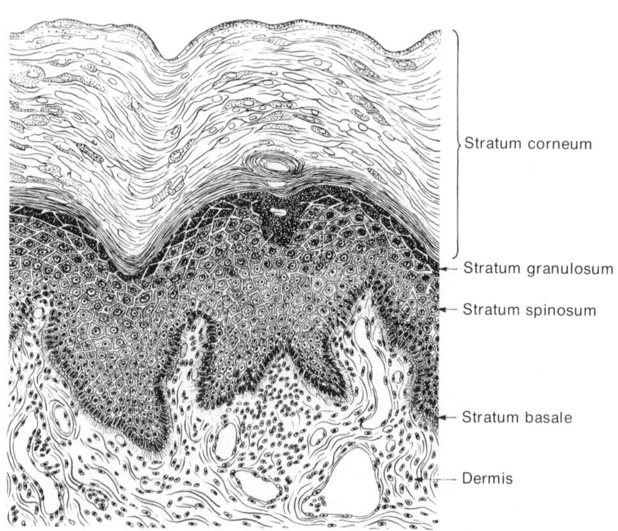

Figure 112. Epidermis. (After W. Bargmann, 1967.)

Melanocytes

Scattered between the keratinocytes of the basal layer are the melanocytes, which can be better visualized by special stains. Thin cytoplasmic processes extend between the adjacent keratinocytes. The melanocytes synthesize melanin.

Under the influence of an enzyme synthesized by melanocytes (tyrosinase), tyrosine oxidizes into dopa, and dopa-quinone, which, after several other oxidations and polymerization, forms melanin. Through histochemical tests (the dopa reaction), tyrosinase activity of the melanocytes can be localized. Stages of melanin synthesis by melanocytes may be studied microscopically. Synthesis of tyrosinase takes place in the granular endoplasmic reticulum. The Golgi complex isolates the aggregate enzyme molecules in vesicles, which become premelanosomes. These are small, ovoid organelles enveloped by a membrane and containing an inner membrane system in which tyrosinase molecules are aligned. Oxidation of tyrosine by the tyrosinase molecules causes melanin to appear on the inner membranes of the premelanosomes. When melanin deposition is complete, the premelanosomes become known as melanosomes. These are the true secretory granules of melanin.

The intensity of skin pigmentation depends on the amount of melanin synthesized by the melanocytes, not on the number of melanocytes.

Langerhans Cells

Langerhans cells are scattered between the keratinocytes of the stratum spinosum. They are distinguished from melanocytes only via electron microscopy. The cytoplasm is free premelanosomes and melanosomes, but small discoid quasi-specific organelles are prominent (Langerhans granules). The nature, origin, and role of Langerhans cells and their discoid granules are unknown. Some authors postulate a mesenchymal origin and a macrophagic role.

II. Dermis (Corium)

The dermis is a connective tissue, usually loose at the periphery and more dense (fibrous) in the deeper portions. It contains numerous blood and lymph vessels, nerves, and free sensory and corpuscular nerve endings, as well as various cutaneous appendages extending from the epidermis into the dermis (pilosebaceous follicles and sweat glands).

III. Hypodermis

The hypodermis is a continuation of the dermis. It is a highly vascularized loose connective tissue, which, depending on nutritional conditions and areas of the body, contains varying amounts of adipose tissue.

B. SKIN APPENDAGES

I. Sweat (Sudoriferous) Glands

These are exocrine glands, simple tubes bundled together, secreting sweat. Their secretory portion (simple cuboidal epithelium) is surrounded by myoepithelial cells in the deep dermis. Excretory ducts (bistratified cuboidal epithelium) coil towards the surface of the epidermis. Sweat glands have a segmental sympathetic innervation.

II. Pilosebaceous Follicles

Hairs

Hairs develop from a tubular invagination of the epidermis, which invades the dermis. This epidermal invagination, constituting the epithelial sheath of the hair, thickens at its deep extremity and forms a mass of matrix cells covering a papilla of highly vascularized connective tissue attached to the dermis.

These matrix cells proliferate and give rise to epithelial cells, which become progressively keratinized towards the surface of the skin; thus, the hair shaft is formed in the axis of the epithelial sheath. The quantity and quality of pigment contained in these cells determine the color of the hair.

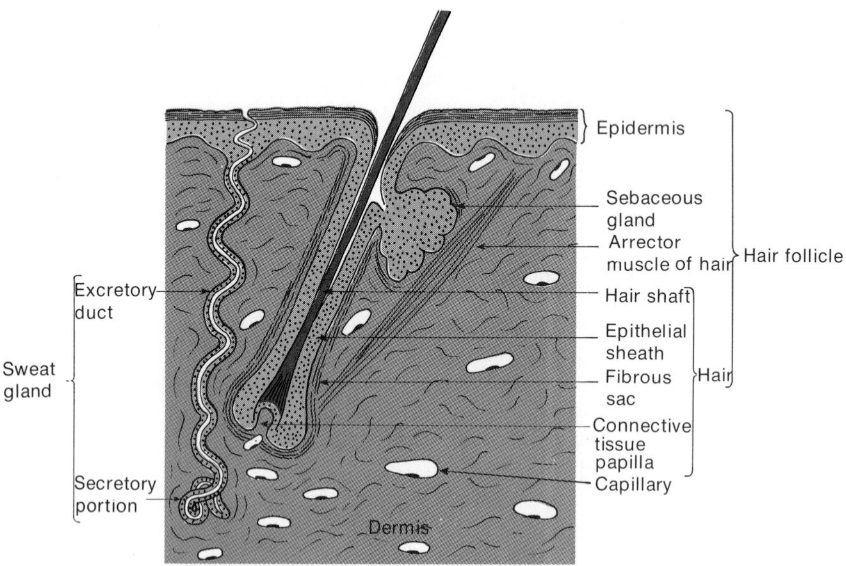

Figure 113. Schematic representation of the principal skin appendages.

The epithelial sheath is surrounded by the "fibrous hair sac," a connective tissue sheath fashioned by the dermis and containing vessels and sensory nerve endings.

Sebaceous Glands

These glands (exocrine, simple alveolar, holocrine) secrete a lipid product, sebum. They are appendages of hairs, with secretory portions made up of one or several saccular alveoli whose walls are of cuboidal epithelium. Inside are large polyhedral cells, filled with lipid droplets, whose nuclei undergo pyknosis and finally disintegrate. In holocrine secretion the entire cell is eliminated along with its contents. A single, short excretory duct opens at the epithelial sheath of hair.

Arrector Pili

This muscle is a small smooth muscle with segmental sympathetic innervation. Its contraction (in response to cold, fear, and so forth) sets off the erection of hair ("goose pimples").

III. Nails

Nails are made of closely compacted horny scales, residues of keratinized epithelial cells. They arise through tangential proliferation of the nail matrix, and grow continually, since desquamation does not occur.

C. TOPOGRAPHIC FEATURES

I. Thin or "Smooth" Skin

All skin, with the exception of that of the palmar surface of hands and fingers, and plantar surface of the feet and toes, is called "smooth" because of a thin epidermal layer (although the thickness of dermis and hypodermis may vary). It contains small or moderate numbers of sweat glands as well as pilosebaceous follicles. The surface lacks ridges and grooves and forms only a small checkered network of lines between the slightly depressed orifices of the pilosebaceous follicles.

Some portions of "smooth" skin are distinguished by: (1) density or caliber and length of hairs (scalp, eyebrows, mustache, beard, external genitalia, and so forth); (2) presence of sweat glands (lips, glans, inner side of the prepuce, labia minora, and so forth); or (3) presence of "apocrine" sweat glands. The latter differ from the usual sweat glands (called "eccrine") by: (a) their limitation to certain portions of the body (underarm, pubis, anal region, areola and nipple, prepuce and scrotum, labia minora, and so forth); (b) the nature of the secretory product (thicker, more odoriferous, and richer in lipids and pigments than normal sweat); and (c) their variations in function depending on stages in reproductive life. The ceruminal glands of the external ear canal are a special variety of apocrine sweat glands.

II. "Thick" Skin

Thick skin is characteristic of the palms of the hands, the fingers, the soles of the feet, and the toes. It presents, point by point, the opposite characteristics of the so-called smooth skin: (1) thickness of the epidermis is considerable, (2) there are abundant sweat glands, (3) there are no pilosebaceous follicles, and (4) grooves and ridges (fingerprints) are visible with the naked eye, formed by dermal papillae in the dermis. In the epidermis these are obvious as ridges separated by grooves. The orifices of sweat gland ducts open at the top of these ridges. The pattern formed by these ridges and grooves is unique for each individual and inalterable (hence their utilization for identification purposes). It should be noted that thick skin contains numerous arteriovenous anastomoses in the dermis and hypodermis.

II. THE EYE

To reach the visual retina, light rays must traverse the transparent media of the eye (in sequence, the cornea, aqueous humor, crystalline lens, and vitreous body). Adjustment of the retinal image formed (accommodation) is mediated by the interplay of the iris (whose opening depends on amount of light) and the lens (whose curvature depends on the distance of the object). The eyeball is covered by a coat of dense, opaque, vascularized fibrous connective tissue (the sclera). It commences at the lateral border of the cornea, with which it is continuous, and is continuous posteriorly with the dura mater of the optic nerve.

A. THE TRANSPARENT MEDIA

I. The Cornea

The cornea is made up of a layer of dense, highly oriented connective tissue that is transparent and avascular; it is covered on both sides by an epithelium (nonkeratinized stratified squamous anteriorly, and simple squamous posteriorly). Nutrition occurs by diffusion from the aqueous humor.

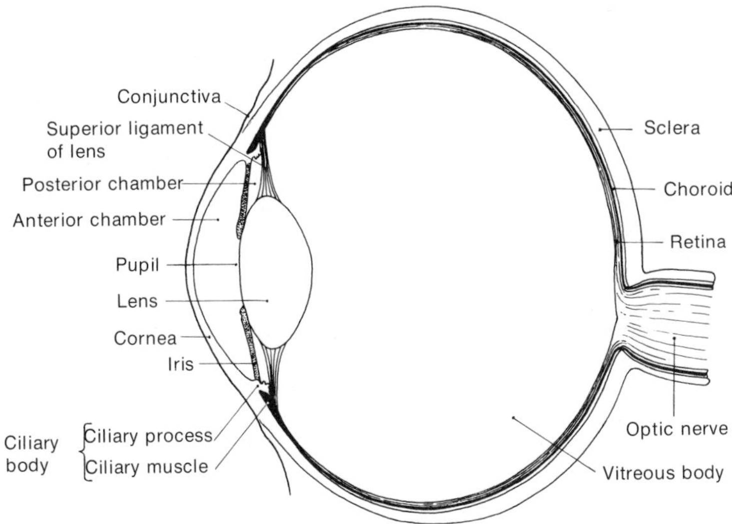

Figure 114. The eyeball (sagittal section). (After Rouviere, 1974.)

II. The Aqueous Humor

The aqueous humor is secreted by ciliary processes which constitute the inner part of the ciliary bodies. These processes are formed from a connective tissue axis rich in vessels and covered by two layers of stratified cuboidal epithelium. This epithelium is the forward prolongation of the visual retina. Its outer layer has the same structure as the pigment epithelium of the visual retina.

After having reached the anterior chamber of the eye, aqueous humor is resorbed, at the irido-corneal angle, by the canal of Schlemm, which opens into the choroidal and scleral veins.

III. Iris

The iris consists of a connective tissue layer that is a continuation of the stroma of the ciliary body. Numerous pigment cells are found here, which determine the color of the eyes. Two layers of smooth muscle are responsible for reflex or synergic variations in the diameter of the pupil: (1) the dilator of the pupil (innervated by the sympathetic nerve), and (2) the constrictor of the pupil (innervated by the parasympathetic nerve). Anteriorly, the iris is covered by a discontinuous layer of fibroblasts and melanocytes. Posteriorly, it is covered by an epithelium identical to that of the ciliary processes.

IV. Crystalline Lens

The crystalline lens is a transparent epithelial body whose cells present three main characteristics: (1) long hexagonal prismatic cells, crowded together, with an anteroposterior axis; (2) an outer nucleated cell layer that contributes to its continued growth; (3) cytoplasm containing specific proteins synthesized during differentiation. Numerous microfilaments appear via electron microscopy.

The lens is suspended from the ciliary body by suspensory ligaments. As a result of contraction of the ciliary muscles in its connective stroma and nervous conduction by the parasympathetic nerve, the lens can modify its shape to accommodate to distance.

V. Vitreous Body

The vitreous body is a viscous transparent substance composed of water, mucopolysaccharides, and collagen. Electron microscopically it appears to be made up of thin filaments distributed within an amorphous ground substance.

B. VISUAL RETINA

From the periphery towards the center of the eyeball, the visual retina consists of four principal types of cells.

I. Pigment Epithelium

This epithelium is made up of a single layer of cuboidal cells containing melanin granules synthesized by them. They send out thin processes that push between the outer segments of the photoreceptors. Pigment epithelium is responsible for nutrition, protection, and isolation of the photoreceptors.

II. Photoreceptors

Except for few small differences, the morphology of the rod and cone cells is identical. From the periphery towards the center of the eyeball, their structural features include:

a. *The outer segment,* elongated and cylindrical for the rods, shorter and conical for the cones. This portion is stacked with flattened membranous discs, containing the visual pigments (rhodopsin in the rod cells, iodopsin in the cone cells).

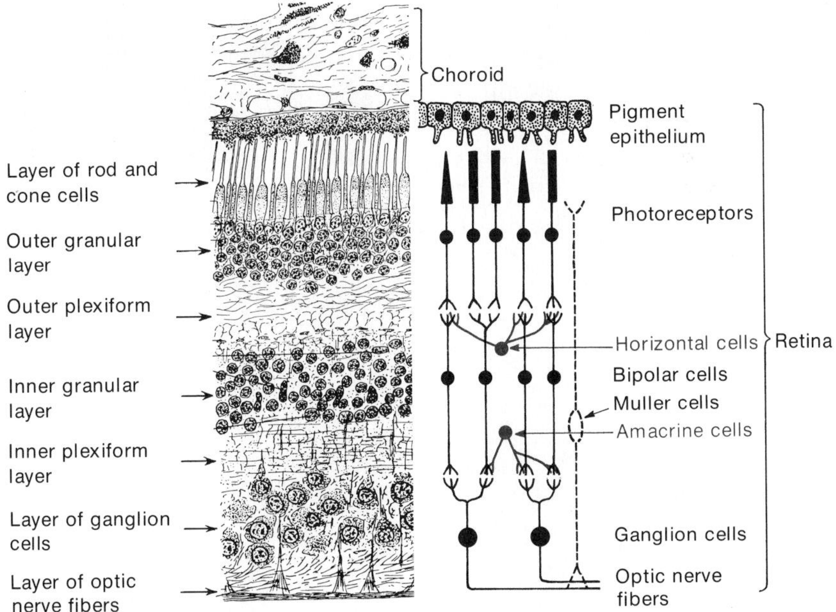

Figure 115. Schematic representation of a section of the retina. *Left,* As seen with the optic microscope (×360) (after O. Bucher, 1972); *right,* cellular schema.

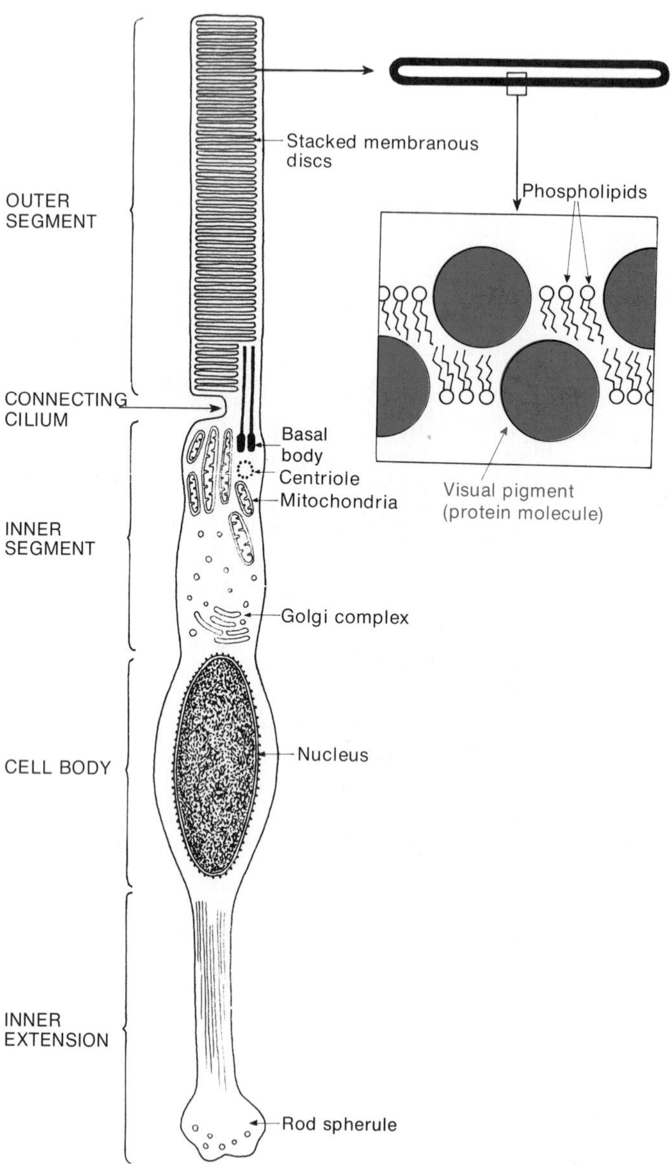

Figure 116. The general structure of a photoreceptor.

b. *The inner segment,* which gives rise to the connecting stalk, contains a centriole, numerous mitochondria, and an extensive Golgi complex.

c. *The cell body,* with its central nucleus.

d. *The inner extension,* thin and variable in length, ends in a rod spherule or cone pedicle making contact with dendrites of the bipolar cells.

These photoreceptor cells are responsible for the transformation of light quanta into nerve impulses. Under the action of absorbed light, visual pigment molecules alter their configuration (isomerization of 11-*cis* retinal to *trans* retinal). Through this modification, depolarization of the cell membrane and formation of action potentials (nerve impulses) are achieved.

III. Bipolar Cells

From the cell body, which contains the nucleus, an external extension (dendrite) forms a synaptic junction with the presynaptic ganglia of the photoreceptors; an inner extension (axon) likewise branches out and makes synaptic contact with the ganglion cells. One bipolar cell synapses with only one cone and one ganglion cell, but other bipolar cells connect to several rods. Each ganglion cell synapses with several bipolar cells. It is for this reason that visual acuity is better at the fovea centralis (containing only cones) than at the periphery of the retina (where rods predominate).

IV. Ganglion Cells

The cell body of ganglion cells is large and contains a large nucleus. Their dendrites synapse with the axon of the bipolar cells, and their very long axon penetrates the optic nerve, where it becomes myelinated.

In addition to these four cell types, the retina contains connecting neurons (horizontal cells and amacrine cells), which form junctions between photoreceptors, and between bipolar cells and ganglion cells. Glial cells (Müller cells), lying perpendicular to the surface of the retina over most of its thickness, fill the spaces between the nerve elements with their cytoplasmic processes.

Nutrition of the peripheral layers of the retina (pigment epithelium and photoreceptors) occurs via capillaries of the choroid (loose connective tissue, highly vascularized, and situated between the deep layer of the sclera and the surface layer of the retina). Other layers are nourished by retinal capillaries (springing from the branches of the central artery of the retina), which circulate in that part of the retina close to its deep surface.

C. ACCESSORIES OF THE EYEBALL

The *lacrimal glands* (exocrine, tubulo-acinous, and of the serous type) secrete tears.

The eyelids, which are sheets of connective tissue covered anteriorly by the epidermis and posteriorly by the conjunctiva, contain the orbicularis oculi muscle of the eyelids and the meibomian glands (large sebaceous glands not appended to hairs). Lashes are attached at their outer edge, which bears the orifices of excretory ducts of numerous small sweat glands and sebaceous glands.

The conjunctiva is a mucosa of stratified columnar epithelium containing some goblet cells. It covers the anterior part of the sclera (corresponding to the "white of the eye"), and is reflected at the posterior side of the eyelids.

III. THE EAR

A. GENERAL STRUCTURE

I. External Ear

The auricle, external auditory meatus, and the tympanic membrane are covered by skin. Cerumen is the secretory product of ceruminous glands (a variety of apocrine sweat glands) and of sebaceous glands, located in the dermis covering the external auditory meatus.

II. Middle Ear

The ossicles (malleus, incus, and stapes), the inner side of the tympanic membrane, the bony walls of the tympanic cavity, and mastoid cavities are covered by a thin mucosa. This squamous or cuboidal epithelium contains some islets of ciliated cells and some mucous or seromucous glandular cells.

The tympanic membrane consists of an outer epithelium (epidermis) and an inner epithelium (of the ear drum) separated by a fibrous lamina containing the manubrium of the malleus.

The mucosa of the auditory tube consists of a respiratory type of epithelium. Its outer portion rests on a cartilaginous and fibrous base, while its deeper portion rests on bone.

III. Internal Ear

The membranous labyrinth is a closed cavity bounded by an epithelium containing endolymph. It develops in early embryonic life as a spherical body (from invagination of the otic vesicle). During development, unequal proliferation transforms it into a progressively more complicated system by the formation of bulges, constrictions, and elongations of some portions. At the end, several distinctive but intercommunicating parts can be recognized: utricle, saccule, semicircular ducts, and ducts and sacs of the endolymphatic system, as well as the cochlear duct. Later, the simple squamous or cuboidal epithelium of the membranous labyrinth differentiates into (1) the sensory receptor zones (maculae of the utricle and saccule, crista ampullaris of the semicircular ducts, and organ of Corti) and (2) the stria vascularis, secreting endolymph, and the endolymphatic sac which resorbs it. As the site of endolymph production, the stratified stria vascularis is characterized by the presence of blood capillaries between epithelial cells. This is the only epithelium conveying blood vessels. The endolymphatic sac, a blind end of the endolymphatic duct, is bound by simple columnar epithelium, consisting of cells with long microvilli and numerous pinocytotic vesicles.

Mesenchymal differentiation forms the *bony labyrinth* around the membranous labyrinth. The two are separated by perilymphatic spaces containing perilymph. Thus, the bony vestibule houses the saccule, utricle, and semicircular canals. The aqueduct of the vestibule contains the endolymphatic canals and sac. The cochlea contains the cochlear duct, resembling a snail shell with a conical bony axis, the modiolus. Around this a bony tube makes two-and-three-quarter spiral turns. The bony canal is divided length-

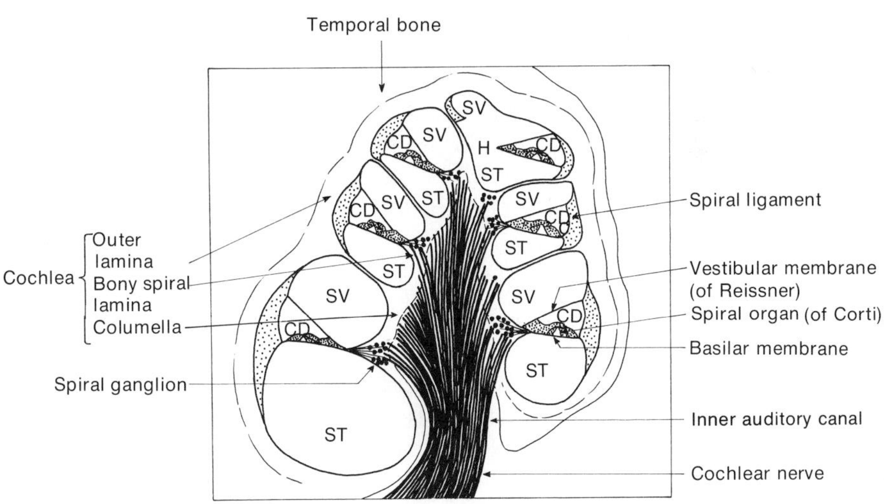

Figure 117. Longitudinal section of the cochlea. *CD,* Cochlear duct; *SV,* Scala vestibuli; *ST,* Scala tympani; *H,* Helicotrema. (After J. Poirier and J. Chevreau: Feuillets d'Histologie. Paris, Maloine, 1971.)

wise into two compartments by a bony spiral lamina inserted on the modiolus, containing the spiral ganglion (of Corti). This is continuous laterally with the basilar membrane inserted on the spiral ligament. These two compartments, comprising a lower cavity (scala tympani) and an upper cavity (scala vestibuli), communicate with each other through a small orifice (helicotrema) located at the apex of the cochlea. The cochlear canal forms a spiral between those two scalae. In cross section it is seen to be roughly triangular, with its inner side differentiated into the spiral organ of Corti. This rests on the basilar membrane separating it from the scala tympani. The outer surface of the cochlear duct is differentiated into a stria vascularis, resting against the upper part of the spiral ligament. The superior surface constitutes (together with flattened, perilymphatic mesenchymal cells) the vestibular membrane of Reissner, which separates it from the scala vestibuli.

B. VESTIBULAR AND AUDITORY ZONES OF SENSORY RECEPTION

I. Maculae of the Utricle and Saccule

The maculae (one of the utricle, the other in the saccule) contain vestibular sensory cells of type I and type II (see page 214), which are scattered in a layer of supporting cells. The otolithic membrane (layer of a gelatinous ground substance containing fascicles of thin fibrils and, in the upper part, small masses of calcium carbonate, the otoliths) rests with its deep face on apical microvilli of the sensory cells. Afferent (vestibular nerve) and efferent nerve endings surround the base of the sensory cells. The maculae are stimulated by inclination of the head. In fact, when the position of the head changes, the otoliths by reason of their weight push against the microvilli of sensory cells. Their distortion stimulates the afferent vestibular nerve fibers.

II. Crista Ampullaris of the Semicircular Canals

The crista ampullaris of the semicircular canals resembles the maculae in basic structure; however, its shape is different and the cupula contains no otoliths. The crista ampullaris is stimulated by movements of the head with an induced flow of endolymph in the semicircular canals.

III. Organ of Corti

At the center of the organ of Corti is the tunnel of Corti, which is triangular in cross section. The outer and inner walls are constituted respec-

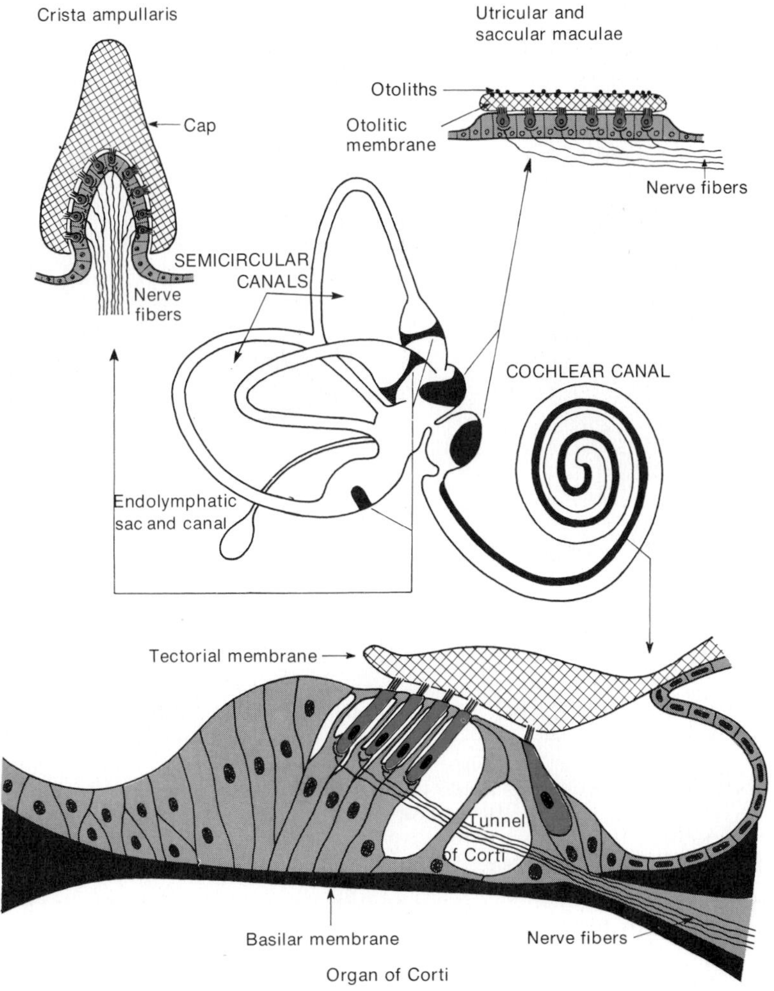

Figure 118. Schematic representation of the membranous labyrinth and sensory receptor zones. Sensory cells are shown in red, supporting cells in gray.

tively by a row of outer pillar cells and a row of inner pillar cells. These are supporting cells, containing large amounts of tonofibrils in their cytoplasm. On each side of this tunnel is an arrangement of sensory cells supported by the "cells of Deiters." Externally there are three or four rows of outer sensory cells, and internally one row of inner sensory cells. The basal pole of the cells of Deiters rests on the basilar membrane, and their upper part surrounds the base of the sensory cells and adjacent nerve endings. They send out a long process whose flattened upper extremity ("phalange") contributes, together with its homologues and the phalanges of the pillar cells, to the formation of the "reticular membrane." This membrane surrounds and

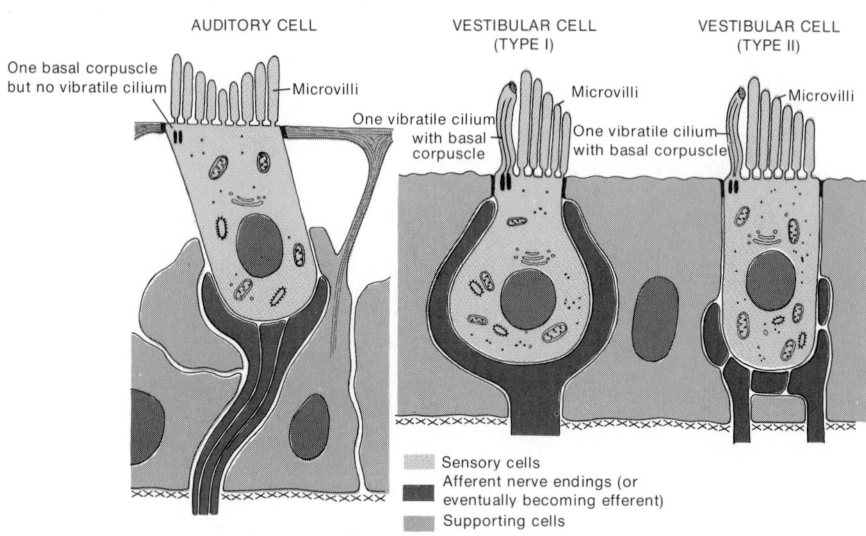

Figure 119. Sensory cells of the inner ear.

TABLE 31. Sensory Zones of the Inner Ear

Vestibular and Auditory Zones of Sensory Reception of the Inner Ear			Sensory Nerves Leaving From These Sites
Name	*Constituents*	*Localization*	
MACULAE	Vestibular sensory cells of types I and II Supporting cells Otolithic membrane	Utricle Saccule	Vestibular nerve (equilibrium)
CRISTA AMPULLARIS	Vestibular sensory cells of types I and II Supporting cells Cupula	Ampulla of the outer semicircular canal Ampulla of the upper semicircular canal Ampulla of the posterior semicircular canal	
SPIRAL ORGAN OF CORTI	Auditory sensory cells Supporting cells Tectorial membrane	Cochlear canal	Cochlear nerve (audition)

maintains the apical pole of the sensory cells. On each side of these cells, two bodies of supporting cells are continuous with the epithelium covering the bulge of the spiral ligament and with the epithelium of the stria vascularis. From this is formed the tectorial membrane (fibrillar in nature) which comes to lie on the microvilli of the sensory cells.

Sound vibrations stimulate the auditory sensory cells via oscillations of the basilar membrane. These vibrations cause displacement of the outer pillar cells; since the tectorial membrane does not move, the apical microvilli of the sensory cells are distorted, setting off the stimulus.

IV. Vestibular and Auditory Sensory Cells

The vestibular and auditory zones of sensory reception show extensive similarities in their general structure. The microvilli on the apical poles of the sensory cells are covered by the tectorial membrane, otolithic membrane, or cupula, whose relative shifting is the source of the stimulus. The basal poles of these cells are in contact with afferent nerve fibers. Thus, sensory cells conduct sensory information to the central nervous system. Supporting cells surround the sensory cells and nerve endings in a variable manner.

The ultrastructure of sensory cells, as well as their close relationship with nerve endings, permits distinction of three cell types: vestibular sensory cells of type I; vestibular sensory cells of type II; and auditory sensory cells. The chief characteristics are represented schematically in Figure 119. Essential common points should be noted: microvilli with thin bases, presence of a cilium or ciliary residue in the form of a basal corpuscle, contacts with afferent nerve endings, and closely enveloping supporting cells.

IV. OLFACTORY MUCOSA

The olfactory mucosa covers a very small area at the posterosuperior part of each nasal cavity. Its pseudostratified columnar epithelium (with basal cells and supporting cells) has fusiform olfactory neurosensory cells. The dendritic peripheral processes end at the epithelial surface in a small spherical bulge covered by cilia. The axonal processes enter the lamina propria, where they invaginate into Schwann cells. They form nonmyelinated nerve nets which traverse the cribriform plate of the ethmoid bone and end in the olfactory bulb. The lamina propria contains sensitive nerve endings, numerous blood vessels, and large mucous glands, whose secretory ducts open onto the surface of the epithelium (Bowman's glands) (see Fig. 61).

The essential mechanisms of odor perception are not well known. Odoriferous molecules contacting the olfactory epithelium during inspiration and expiration are absorbed at the surface of the cellular membrane of the cilia of sensory cells. Absorption is a reversible physicochemical phenomenon involving a mucous film secreted by the mucous (Bowman's) glands. The contact achieved by selective absorption (necessitating a steric compatibility between odoriferous molecules and cell membrane) is accompanied by a depolarization of the membrane of the sensory cell, setting off nerve messages along the fibers of the olfactory nerve.

V. TASTE BUDS

Taste buds, located in the epithelium of the fungiform and circumvallate papillae on the back of the tongue, are ovoid formations made of about 20 fusiform cells arranged in parallel. They reach the surface of the epithelium at the level of the taste pores. These cells consist of supporting cells and sensory cells transmitting taste information to the nerve endings (of the glossopharyngeal and facial nerve) (see Fig. 68).

Bibliography

1. Andrew W. *Microfabric of Man. A textbook of histology.* Yearbook Medical Publishers, Chicago, 1966.
2. Arey L. B. *Human Histology.* 4th Ed. W. B. Saunders Co., Philadelphia, 1974.
3. Bargmann W. *Histologie und mikroskopische Anatomie des Menschen.* 6th Ed. Georg Thieme Verlag, Stuttgart, 1967.
4. Bloom W. and Fawcett D. W. *Textbook of Histology.* 10th Ed. W. B. Saunders Co., Philadelphia, 1975.
5. Bucher O. *Diagnostic et diagnostic différential en cytologie et en histologie normales.* Masson et Cie., Paris, 1973.
6. Cruickshank B., Dodds T. D. and Gardner D. L. *Human Histology.* 2nd ed. E. and S. Livingstone, Edinburgh, 1968.
7. Czyba J. C. and Girod C. *Cours d'histologie et embryologie.* 2 Vols. Simep, Villeurbanne, 1972.
8. Elias H. and Pauly J. E. *Human Microanatomy.* 3rd Ed. F. A. Davis Co., Philadelphia, 1966.
9. Girod C. and Czyba J. C. *Cours sur la biologie de la reproduction.* 2 Vols. Simep, Villeurbanne, 1972.
10. Greep R. O. *Histology.* 2nd Ed. McGraw-Hill Book Co., New York, 1966.
11. Ham A. W. *Histology.* 5th Ed. J. B. Lippincott, Philadelphia, 1965.
12. *Hewer's Textbook of Histology for Medical Students* (revised by S. Bradbury). 9th Ed. W. Heinemann, London, 1969.
13. Leeson T. S. and Leeson C. R. *Histology.* 3rd Ed. W. B. Saunders Co., Philadelphia, 1976.
14. Poirier J. and Chevreau J. *Feuillets d'histologie humaine.* 8 fascicules. Maloine, Paris.

    Fascicule 1: *Épithéliums de revêtement; glandes; tissu conjonctif; cartilage et os* (2nd Ed., 1972).

    Fascicule 2: *Tissus musculares; tissu nerveaux; sang* (2nd Ed., 1972).

    Fascicule 3: *Appareil cardio-vasculaire; vasseaux lymphatiques; organes hématopoïétiques et lymphoïdes; appareil respiratore* (2nd Ed., 1972).

    Fascicule 4: *Tube digestif; foie et voies biliaires; pancréas exocrine* (2nd Ed., 1972).

Fascicule 5: *Appareil urinaire; appareil génital masculin; appareil génital féminin* (2nd Ed., 1972).
Fascicule 6: *Hypophyse; thyroïde; parathyroïde; surrénales; pancréas endocrine* (2nd Ed., 1972).
Fascicule 7: *Peau et phanerès; seins; organes des sens* (1971).
Fascicule 8: *Neurohistologie* (1972).

Atlases

15. BERGMAN R. A. et AFIFI A. K. *Atlas of Microscopic Anatomy.* W. B. Saunders Co., Philadelphia, 1974.
16. COUJARD R. and COUJARD-CHAMPY C. *Atlas de traveaux pratiques d'histologie.* 2. fascicules. Vigot, Paris.
    Fascicule 1: *Les tissus* (1964).
    Fascicule 2: *Les organes* (1965).
17. DALION J. *Planches et diapositives d'histologie (366 diapositives présentées en 24 depliants).* Maloine, Paris, 1972.
18. Di Fiore M. S. H. *Atlas of Human Histology.* 3rd Ed. Lea and Febiger, Philadelphia, 1968.

Index

Page numbers in *italics* refer to illustrations; (t) indicates tables.